Weight Regulation and Curing Acquired Obesity

Weight Regulation and Curing Acquired Obesity

Gary Horndeski, MD

CHI St. Luke's Health — Brazosport Hospital
Lake Jackson, Texas
United States

Elisa Gonzalez, PA-C

CHI St. Luke's Health — Brazosport Hospital
Lake Jackson, Texas
United States

ELSEVIER

Elsevier
Radarweg 29, PO Box 211, 1000 AE Amsterdam, Netherlands
The Boulevard, Langford Lane, Kidlington, Oxford OX5 1GB, United Kingdom
50 Hampshire Street, 5th Floor, Cambridge, MA 02139, United States

Notices
Knowledge and best practice in this field are constantly changing. As new
research and experience broaden our understanding, changes in research
methods, professional practices, or medical treatment may become necessary.

Practitioners and researchers must always rely on their own experience and
knowledge in evaluating and using any information, methods, compounds, or
experiments described herein. In using such information or methods they
should be mindful of their own safety and the safety of others, including
parties for whom they have a professional responsibility.

To the fullest extent of the law, neither the Publisher nor the authors,
contributors, or editors, assume any liability for any injury and/or damage to
persons or property as a matter of products liability, negligence or otherwise,
or from any use or operation of any methods, products, instructions, or ideas
contained in the material herein.

Library of Congress Cataloging-in-Publication Data
A catalog record for this book is available from the Library of Congress

British Library Cataloguing-in-Publication Data
A catalogue record for this book is available from the British Library

ISBN: 978-0-323-77854-1

> For information on all Elsevier publications visit our website
> at https://www.elsevier.com/books-and-journals

Publisher: Cathleen Sether
Acquisitions Editor: Belinda Kuhn
Editorial Project Manager: Sam W. Young
Production Project Manager: Kiruthika Govindaraju
Cover Designer: Alan Studholme

Working together
to grow libraries in
developing countries

www.elsevier.com • www.bookaid.org

Typeset by TNQ Technologies

Dedicated to Henry S. Koopman and all the other researchers who's work provided the scientific basis for this book.

Contents

Preface

Ten percent of all healthcare cost in America is directly or indirectly related to obesity. Eighteen percent of the gross national product is consumed in healthcare. In 2018, approximately 369 billion dollars were spent on obesity. Currently, there are 14 medical journals with obesity in the title listed in the US National Library of Medicine. Despite the huge cost of obesity and extensive research, there is no unified theory of weight regulation or an explanation for the rising incidence of obesity. The most effective therapy for obesity has been surgical. Gastric restriction or intestinal malabsorption operations have been performed despite the fact that no one has hypothesized that gastric enlargement or increased intestinal absorption creates obesity. The purpose of this book is to present a unified theory of weight regulation, explain the pathology of acquired obesity, and offer therapy directed to correct the underlying pathophysiology.

Acknowledgment

Thanks to the Moody Medical Library of the University of Texas at Galveston for allowing us to use their facility, and the librarians who assisted us, especially Anne Howard. Also, thanks to Jana Reed for the many rewrites and figures.

The basics

Chapter outline

Abstract

Obesity is mathematically defined as a body mass index (BMI) of greater than or equal to 30 kg per meter squared. BMI is a physical measurement that corresponds to pressure. Obesity results from the accumulation of the ingested fat when the caloric intake exceeds caloric expenditure. One pound of fat stores 3500 kilocalories of potential energy and occupies 0.5 L. Fat has a fixed distribution throughout the body that is dependent on age, sex, and genetics. The distribution ratio D is defined as intra-abdominal fat volume divided by total fat volume. Fat weight can be sensed indirectly by sensing fat volume.

Keywords: Body mass index; Fat distribution ratio D; Fat weight energy volume triad; Obesity; Sensing; Weight regulation.

Mathematics is the language of science. Determining numeric values allows mathematical analysis, which facilitates solving complex problems. Obesity is a chronic disease of increasing prevalence and severity. Unlike diabetes, obesity is defined by physical measurements, not a biochemical test. Obesity is mathematically defined as a body mass index (BMI) of greater than or equal to 30 kilograms per meter squared (Table 1.1). BMI can also be calculated by the formula BMI equals 704 times pounds divided by inches squared (Table 1.2). The units of BMI correspond to pressure, which is a physical measurement. Meter squared is two dimensional and corresponds to surface area. However, the BMI formula uses height squared, not body surface area. In adults, height does not significantly change, therefore BMI change is weight dependent. In growing children, height increases which can reduce BMI. Weight is composed

Table 1.1 BMI classification.

		Underweight	<18.5
18.5	≤	Normal	<25
25	≤	Overweight	<30
30	≤	Obese	<40
40	≤	Extreme obese	

Table 1.2 Body Mass Index table.

BMI / Height	17	18	19	20	21	22	23	24	25	26	27	28	29	30	31	32	33	34	35	36
4'10	81	86	91	96	100	105	110	115	119	124	129	134	138	143	148	153	158	162	167	172
4'11	84	89	94	99	104	109	114	119	124	128	133	138	143	148	153	158	163	168	173	178
5'	87	92	97	102	107	112	118	123	128	133	138	143	148	153	158	163	168	174	179	184
5'1	90	95	100	106	111	116	122	127	132	137	143	148	153	158	164	169	174	180	185	190
5'2	93	98	104	109	115	120	126	131	136	142	147	153	158	164	169	175	180	186	191	197
5'3	96	101	107	113	118	124	130	135	141	146	152	158	163	169	175	180	186	191	197	203
5'4	99	105	110	116	122	128	134	140	145	151	157	163	169	174	180	186	192	197	204	209
5'5	102	108	114	120	126	132	138	144	150	156	162	168	174	180	186	192	198	204	210	216
5'6	105	111	118	124	130	136	142	148	155	161	167	173	179	186	192	198	204	210	216	223
5'7	108	115	121	127	134	140	146	153	159	166	172	178	185	191	198	204	211	217	223	230
5'8	112	118	125	131	138	144	151	158	164	171	177	184	190	197	203	210	216	223	230	236
5'9	115	122	128	135	142	149	155	162	169	176	182	189	196	203	209	216	223	230	236	243
5'10	118	125	132	139	146	153	160	167	174	181	188	195	202	209	216	222	229	236	243	251
5'11	122	129	136	143	150	157	165	172	179	186	193	200	208	215	222	229	236	243	250	258
6'	125	133	140	147	154	162	169	177	184	191	199	206	213	221	228	235	242	250	258	265
6'1	129	136	144	151	159	166	174	182	189	197	204	212	219	227	235	242	250	257	265	272
6'2	132	140	148	155	163	171	179	186	194	202	210	218	225	233	241	249	256	264	272	280
6'3	135	144	152	160	168	176	184	192	200	208	216	224	232	240	248	256	264	272	279	288
6'4	139	148	156	164	172	180	189	197	205	213	221	230	238	246	254	263	271	279	287	295
6'5	143	152	160	168	177	185	193	202	210	219	227	235	244	253	261	270	278	286	295	303
6'6	147	156	164	173	181	190	199	207	216	225	233	241	250	259	268	277	285	294	302	311

Body Mass Index Table

of two components: lean body weight and fat weight. Lean body weight refers to nonfat weight and is stable unless growth or changes in bone or muscle mass occur. Since lean body weight is stable, obesity occurs from excessive accumulation of fat. Obesity does not change height but does change volume. Since volume is three dimensional and the vertical dimension is fixed, then one or both of the horizontal dimensions must increase. Does acquired obesity create horizontal expansion or does horizontal expansion create acquired obesity?

Energy is required to sustain life and is derived from three major food components: protein, carbohydrate, and fat. Protein is required for cell growth and maintenance. Excess dietary protein cannot be converted into fat, is not excreted, nor stored as an energy source but is consumed. Unlike protein, carbohydrate can be stored as an energy source. The average man of 154 pounds (70 kg) has 0.2 pounds of carbohydrate stored in the liver and 1.1 pounds in muscles. The 1.3 pounds of carbohydrate store 2400 kilocalories (Kcals), which will supply the energy requirements for about 1 day, based on a 2600 Kcals per day diet for males or 1900 Kcals for females. Medical research has shown that carbohydrate conversion into fat is limited to a maximum of 5 grams per day, even in people consuming 500 g of carbohydrate per day.[1,2] Excess carbohydrates can neither be excreted nor be stored beyond the previously described limits, and conversion into fat is extremely limited. Elevated carbohydrate levels in the blood activate the pancreas to secrete insulin which drives carbohydrates into the cells, where they are consumed as an energy source. People frequently sense this as a sugar rush.

Fat is required for survival and is composed of essential and nonessential fats. Essential fats are acquired from the diet and cannot be synthesized by the body. Unlike protein or carbohydrate, dietary fat can be stored in large quantities, when caloric intakes exceed expenditure. An excess of 3500 Kcals is required for 1 pound of fat storage, which occupies 0.5 L (Fig.1.1). When dietary caloric intake is less than caloric expenditure, fat is removed from storage. Removal of one pound of stored fat releases 3500 Kcals. The fat in our body represents a lifetime accumulation from caloric excess. The average man of 154 pounds has 20 pounds of fat stored in adipose tissue, plus 1 pound stored in the liver, and 0.6 pounds stored in muscles. Adipose tissue has a fixed distribution throughout the body that is determined by age, sex, and genetics. The volume of intra-abdominal fat, divided by the total volume of fat, is defined as the distribution ratio, D, Eq.(1.1) Intra-abdominal adipose tissue is metabolically more active than extraabdominal adipose tissue and the volume changes faster. Men have a higher percent of intra-abdominal adipose tissue than women, especially in the upper abdomen around the stomach and omentum.[3] Obese men are apple shaped and obese women are pear shaped due to fat distribution.

$$\text{Distribution Ratio } D = \frac{\text{Intra-abdominal Fat Volume}}{\text{Total Fat Volume}} \qquad (1.1)$$

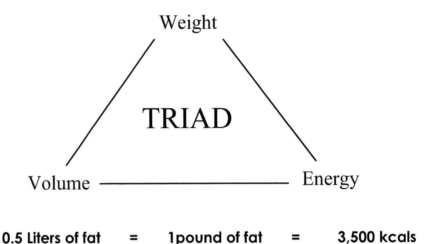

0.5 Liters of fat   =   1 pound of fat   =   3,500 kcals

FIGURE 1.1

The volume, weight and energy triad.

I weigh 172 pounds and over the past 30 years my weight has fluctuated ± 3 pounds or ±1.7%. Consuming 2600 Kcals per day for 30 years required 28,470,000 Kcals. My weight varied ±3 pounds which corresponded to 3500 Kcals x 3 or ±10,500 Kcals. Over a 30-year period, my caloric intake balanced caloric expenditure (±10,500 Kcals/ 28,470,000 Kcals = ±0.00037) within ±0.037%. Weight regulation and energy balance this precise could only be achieved by an internal control system. Since fat weight, fat energy and fat volume have a fixed mathematical relationship, a control system that regulates any one of them, regulates all three of them. For a control system to regulate, it must be capable of sensing. For example, blood pressure is regulated by pressure sensing receptors in the aortic arch and carotid sinus. The question is can fat weight, fat energy, or fat volume be sensed? Weight is the force generated by the earth and is equal to mass times gravity. Experiments performed by NASA on the international space station, in zero gravity, have shown that astronauts do not gain weight, but lose 1−4 Kg overall. When rats in space return to earth, their weight is identical to control rats that remained on earth.[4] If weight was sensed, then weightlessness should induce hunger and meal volume should increase in an attempt to compensate for weight loss. This has not been observed; therefore, weight is not sensed. Fat stores potential chemical energy but it is not possible to sense potential chemical energy. Neither fat weight nor fat potential chemical energy can be sensed. Can fat volume be sensed?

References

1. Acheson K, Flatt JP, Jequien E. Glycogen synthesis versus lipogenesisafter a 500 gram carbohydrate meal in man. *Metabolism*. 1982;31(12):1234−1240.
2. Acheson K, Schutz Y, Bessard T, Flatt JP, Jequier E. Carbohydrate metabolism and de novo lipogenesis in human obesity. *Am J Clin Nutr*. 1987; 45:78−85.
3. Kotani K, Tokunaga K, Fujioka S, et al. Sexual dimorphism of age-related changes in whole-body fat distribution in the obese. *Int J Obes*. 1994;18: 207−212.
4. Buckey J. *Space Physiology*. New York: Oxford University Press; 2006: 170−171.

Control system theory

Chapter outline

Abstract

There are two types of control systems, open loop and closed loop. Negative feedback inverts a portion of the output and sends it to the input which converts an open loop to a closed loop. Closed loop systems are designed so that the gain of the system depends on the feedback, not the amplification. Weight regulation is achieved by maintaining a constant value of feedback, despite a widely varying fat volume density in the diet. Weight regulation fails and obesity occurs when feedback decreases and the closed loop degenerates and functions similar to an open loop.

Keywords: A dominant; Amplification; F dominant; Fat volume absorption; Fat volume concentration; Gain; Low fat; Medium fat; High fat diet; Negative feedback; Nondominant; Open and closed loop control systems; Reference; Regulation.

The physiology of weight regulation must be elucidated to discover the pathologic changes and the therapy required to cure obesity. Control system theory is taught to engineering students in college but unfortunately not to physicians in medical school. This chapter will provide the information required to understand the mathematical basis of control system theory and weight regulation.

There are two types of controls systems: open loop and closed loop. Open loop control systems have an input I, that is amplified by A, to produce an output O. $I \times A = O$. Fig. 2.1. The gain G of a control system is defined as the output O divided by the input I. Eq. (2.1). An open loop control system can be designed as a regulator to provide a constant

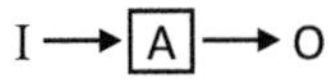

$$I \longrightarrow \boxed{A} \longrightarrow O$$

$$I \times A = O$$

FIGURE 2.1

Open loop.

output O. This is achieved by using an input that is a constant value and is called a reference. Since the input is constant, then the gain G must be constant for the regulator to function and keep the output constant. The gain G of an open loop system is totally dependent on A. If A varies, the control system will not regulate the output.

$$G = \frac{O}{I} = A \tag{2.1}$$

An alternative to the open loop system is the closed loop system. Fig. 2.2. The input I, amplification A, output O, and gain G are identical to an open loop. However, the output is multiplied by the feedback F and is subtracted from the input I. The difference is then multiplied by A to produce O. The gain of the system is determined by Eq. (2.2).

$$
\begin{aligned}
(I - FO) A &= O \\
IA - FOA &= O \\
IA &= O + FOA \\
IA &= O (1 + FA) \\
\frac{A}{1 + FA} &= \frac{O}{I} = G
\end{aligned}
\tag{2.2}
$$

In a closed loop system, the gain is $A/(1 + AF)$. This can be simplified if certain conditions exist. If AF is much greater than 1, then gain is approximately $1/F$. This is called F dominant. We will define $AF \geq 10$ as F dominant. If AF is much less than 1, then gain is approximately A. We will define $AF \leq$ to 0.1 as A dominant. An A dominant system is similar to an open loop system. If neither of these conditions exist, then the system is nondominant.

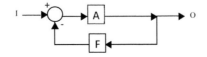

FIGURE 2.2

Closed loop.

Engineers solve complex problems by modeling the problem, writing the appropriate equations and solving them. Since 1 pound of fat occupies 0.5 L of volume, then a volume control system is a weight control system. Volume regulation can be modeled as a closed loop system. The input I is a constant value, the reference volume. Feedback F is intra-abdominal fat volume divided by total fat volume, the distribution ratio D. This has been described in Chapter 1 and is a constant value specific to each patient. The output O is total body fat volume. Amplification A multiplies the volume I minus the volume FO to produce the total fat volume O. A is a number, without units that has three multiplying components. $A = A_C \times A_A \times A_B$. A_C is the volume concentration of fat in the food and is equal to the volume of fat in the food divided by the total volume of food. A_C depends on the diet and the concentration of fat in food varies from 0.0 to 1.00. Table 2.1. All foods have nutritional labels and A_C equals the weight of fat divided by the combined weight of fat plus 0.5 times carbohydrate weight plus 0.7 times protein weight. See Appendix 2.1. The A_C for potato chips is 10 divided by $10 + 7.5 + 1.4$, which equals 0.53 (Appendix 2.2). Fat volume concentration varies exponentially, and we define low fat diet as 0.005 (5×10^{-3}), medium fat diet as 0.05 (5×10^{-2}), and high fat diet as 0.5 (5×10^{-1}). Table 2.2. A_A is the absorption of fat by the intestines and is equal to the volume of fat absorbed divided by the total volume of fat present within the intestines. Humans are 97% efficient in absorbing fat and $A_A = 0.97$ or approximately 1. Medications, diseases, or surgical procedures may also decrease A_A. (The FDA has approved a weight loss drug, Xenical, which results in weight loss by reducing fat absorption by 30%. $A_A = 0.68$ for Xenical). A_B is the amplification determined by the brain that is required to compensate for the fact that the meal volume must be significantly greater than the fat volume deficit. Since A_C is less than or equal to 1 and A_A is less than or equal to 1, then A_B must be significantly greater than 1. This is necessary so that the product $A_C \times A_A \times A_B$ is significantly greater than 1, or the system cannot amplify.

The closed loop control system can be used to model weight regulation. The average male weighs 154 pounds, is 5′7″, BMI is 24.1, and has 20 pounds (10 L) of fat. Studies have shown that intra-abdominal fat is approximately 25% of total fat in males (20% in females), therefore $F = 0.25$.[1] I will assume the control system is F dominant with $AF = 10$, when a medium fat diet is ingested. From these known values and assumptions, the value of $I = 2.75$ and $A = 40$ can be calculated. Fig. 2.3. Using this model, it is possible to predict total fat volume, weight, and BMI with high or low fat diets.

Since A was 40 on a medium fat diet, then A becomes 400 on a high fat diet and 4 on a low fat diet. As a result, the high fat diet is F dominant, $O = 10.8$ L, $W = 156$ pounds, and BMI is 24.4 kg/m^2. The low fat diet is nondominant, $O = 5.5$ L, $W = 144$ pounds, and BMI is 22.6 kg/m^2.

Table 2.1 Fat volume concentration A_C for various foods.

	Food	A_C
Low Fat	Molasses	0.000
	Potatoes	0.001
	Beets	0.001
	Oranges	0.002
	Asparagus	0.002
	Cabbage	0.002
	Tomatoes	0.003
	Spinach	0.003
	Haddock	0.003
	Carrots	0.003
	Peas	0.004
	Apples	0.004
	Strawberries	0.007
Medium Fat	Chicken	0.03
	Bread	0.04
	Milk, fresh, whole	0.043
	Corn	0.047
	Oatmeal, dry	0.081
	Tuna, canned	0.12
High Fat	Lamb, leg	0.20
	Beef	0.24
	Pork, ham	0.34
	Cheese, (cheddar or American)	0.35
	Peanuts	0.48
	Cashew, nuts	0.52
	Chocolate	0.57
	Bacon fat	0.58
	Walnuts, English	0.71
	Bacon fat, broiled	0.84
	Butter	0.89

This model predicts that a 154-pound man's weight will increase 1.2% to 156 pounds on a high fat diet and decreased 6.5% to 144 pound on a low fat diet. A 10,000% fat increase from a low fat to a high fat results in an 8% increase in weight. This model is well regulated and consistent with the clinical observation that normal weight people can consume a high fat diet with minimal weight increase.

The question is how can a control system create obesity? There are only three parameters I, A, and F that determine O. I is a constant

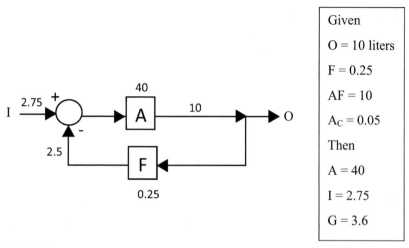

Given
O = 10 liters
F = 0.25
AF = 10
A_C = 0.05
Then
A = 40
I = 2.75
G = 3.6

FIGURE 2.3

Closed loop on average male.

Table 2.2 Fat volume concentration A_C.

0	≤	Low fat 0.005 5×10^{-3}	<0.016
0.016	≤	Medium fat 0.05 5×10^{-2}	<0.16
0.16	≤	High fat 0.5 5×10^{-1}	<1.00

reference level. Increasing I will increase O and can cause obesity. This has been described in medical literature as the set point or fatostat theory.[2] The closed loop control system still functions but obesity is the result of a higher set point, similar to resetting a furnace thermostat to a higher temperature. This is a possible cause of obesity, but most likely is associated with genetic abnormalities, not acquired obesity.

A and F are the only other parameters that can cause obesity. F dominance is required for a closed loop system to regulate output. This requires AF to be much greater than 1. When A decreases, the system is nondominant or A dominant, but a low fat diet cannot increase fat weight. The only alternative is a low F. Obese people like high fat diets and the combination of a high A and a low F can produce obesity.

In my clinical practice, I have a patient that stated "I weigh 240 pounds, but I had weighed this for 20 years. When I go on a diet, I lose 10 to 20 pounds, but my weight always returns to 240 pounds when I stop. What's the point of dieting, if I always return to the same weight?" This patient's obesity persists from the combination of high fat and low F. Even when he decreases his fat 90% from high fat to medium fat, obesity persists. When the product AF is much greater than 1, weight is regulated at a high value (1/F) and obesity persists.

The results of decreasing F from 0.25 to 0 in 10% steps are shown using the average man model in Fig. 2.4. The values of A and I remain the same. The new F values will be used to determine output O, weight, and BMI. Consider F reduced to 30% of the original value (F = 0.25×0.3 = 0.075). When F equals 0.075 and a high fat diet is consumed, the system is F dominant, O = 35.5 L, weight = 205 pounds, and BMI is 32.1 kg/m^2, obese. On a medium fat diet, the system is nondominant, O = 27.5 L, weight = 189 pounds, and BMI is 29.6 kg/m^2, overweight. On a low fat diet, the system is nondominant, O = 8.5 L, weight = 151 pounds, and BMI = 23.7 kg/m^2, normal weight. As a result, decreasing the feedback to 30% of normal increases the weight on all diets. Weight regulation has decreased and is 36% for a 10,000% dietary fat change. Obesity occurs in a high fat diet, overweight occurs in a medium fat diet, and normal weight in a low fat diet.

In Fig. 2.4, when feedback decreases below 28.4% of normal, obesity occurs in both high and medium fat diets. When an obese patient, who normally consumes a high fat diet, decreases his fat intake by 90% to a medium fat diet, obesity persists. This was described in the previous clinical example. With significant loss of feedback, obesity persists despite 90% dietary fat reduction. Only a low fat diet, which requires a 99% reduction from a high fat diet, will produce normal weight. This is usually not accepted by obese people and explains why diets do not cure obesity in people who have significant loss of feedback.

When F equals 0, the closed loop degenerates into an open loop, A dominant system. When F = 0 and a high fat diet is consumed, O = 1100 L, W = 2334 pounds, and BMI is 366 kg/m^2 (weights as high as 1400 pounds has been documented. Other factors such as cardiopulmonary failure prevent greater weights in humans). On a medium fat diet, O = 110 L, W = 354 pounds, and BMI is 55.5 kg/m^2. A low fat diet, O = 11 L, W = 156 pounds, and BMI is 24.5 kg/m^2. Weight regulation is poor and varies 1500% for a 10,000% dietary fat change. The loss of negative feedback results in obesity on medium or high fat diets. Only a low fat diet prevents obesity when feedback is completely lost. Restricting dietary fat can reduce weight and cure obesity, even in complete loss of

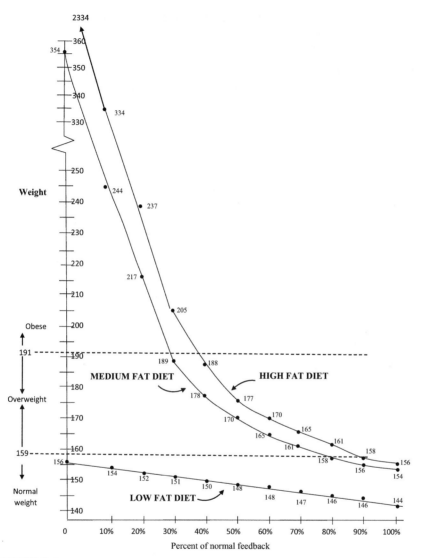

FIGURE 2.4

Percent feedback versus weight for low, medium and high fat diet.

feedback. Unfortunately, obese people will not tolerate low fat diets and will return to their original weight when they return to their original diet.

As a plastic surgeon, I frequently consult patients with complex wounds. On one occasion, I entered the room and saw a bed-ridden, 450-pound man eating high fat food from his bedside table. I asked myself how could he possibly be hungry? After I finished my consult and was about to leave, his brother arrived carrying a shopping bag filled with food. His brother and I stepped outside the room to discuss the patient's condition in private. I asked him why he was enabling this eating disorder. The brother told me he has tried to restrict the patient's access to food at home. This results in the patient crying out in intense pain that requires his brother to acquiesce. I realized that this 450-pound man had lost his negative feedback. Satiety is only achieved during eating, and he experiences almost constant hunger pain.

Appendix 2.1

Determining A_C (fat volume concentration) from a nutritional label.
   Nutritional labels provide the weights of fat, protein, and carbohydrate.

$$\text{Density} \;=\; \frac{\text{Weight}}{\text{Volume}} \qquad D = \frac{W}{V} \quad \text{or} \quad V = \frac{W}{D}$$

$$D_{Fat} \;=\; .9 \text{ g/cm}^3$$

$$D_{Protein} \;=\; 1.35 \text{ g/cm}^3$$

$$D_{Carbohydrate} \;=\; 1.54 \text{ g/cm}^3$$

$$A_C \;=\; \frac{V_{Fat}}{V_{Fat} + V_{Protein} + V_{Carbohydrate}}$$

$$=\; \frac{\dfrac{W_{Fat}}{D_{Fat}}}{\dfrac{W_{Fat}}{D_{Fat}} + \dfrac{W_{Protein}}{D_{Protein}} + \dfrac{W_{Carbohydrate}}{D_{Carbohydrate}}}$$

$$=\; \frac{\dfrac{W_{Fat}}{.9}}{\dfrac{W_{Fat}}{.9} + \dfrac{W_{Protein}}{1.35} + \dfrac{W_{Carbohydrate}}{1.54}}$$

$$=\; \frac{W_{Fat}}{W_{Fat} + \dfrac{.9\,W_{Protein}}{1.35} + \dfrac{.9\,W_{Carbohydrate}}{1.54}}$$

$$=\; \frac{W_{Fat}}{W_{Fat} + .7\,W_{Protein} + .5\,W_{Carbohydrate}}$$

Appendix 2.2

Nutrition Facts

Serving Size 1 oz (28g/About 11 chips)
Servings Per Container About 10

Amount Per Serving

Calories 160   Calories from Fat 90

	% Daily Value*
Total Fat 10g	**16%**
Saturated Fat 1.5g	**7%**
Trans Fat 0g	
Cholesterol 0mg	**0%**
Sodium 70mg	**3%**
Potassium 340mg	**10%**
Total Carbohydrate 15g	**5%**
Dietary Fiber 1g	**5%**
Sugars less than 1g	
Protein 2g	

Vitamin A 0%	•	Vitamin C 10%
Calcium 0%	•	Iron 2%
Vitamin E 6%	•	Thiamin 4%
Niacin 8%	•	Vitamin B_6 10%
Folate 2%	•	Phosphorus 2%

* Percent Daily Values are based on a 2,000 calorie diet. Your daily values may be higher or lower depending on your calorie needs:

		Calories: 2,000	2,500
Total Fat	Less than	65g	80g
Sat Fat	Less than	20g	25g
Cholesterol	Less than	300mg	300mg
Sodium	Less than	2,400mg	2,400mg
Potassium		3,500mg	3,500mg
Total Carbohydrate		300g	375g
Dietary Fiber		25g	30g

Calories per gram:
Fat 9   •   Carbohydrate 4   •   Protein 4

Ingredients: Potatoes, Vegetable Oil (Sunflower, Corn, and/or Canola Oil), and Salt.

Nutritional label from potato chips.

References

1. Kotani K, Tokunaga K, Fujioka S, et al. Sexual dimorphism of age-related changes in whole-body fat distribution in the obese. *Int J Obes*. 1994;18: 207–212.
2. Leibel R. Is obesity due to a heritable difference in 'set point' for adiposity? *West J Med*. 1990;153:429–431.

Satiety

Chapter outline

Abstract

Electronic scales determine weight by mechanical deformation of a strain sensor. Satiety is achieved by a similar mechanism. The stomach wall contains intraganglionic laminar endings (IGLEs) that deform from tension generated by pressure within the stomach wall. Meal volume within the stomach creates gastric wall pressure by the capacity and compliance of the stomach. Intra-abdominal volume (which includes intra-abdominal fat and meal volume) creates intra-abdominal pressure determined by the capacity and compliance of the abdomen. Gastric wall pressure plus intra-abdominal pressure creates tension within the gastric wall by La Place's law. The IGLE cells sense tension generated from both intra-abdominal pressure and gastric wall pressure, producing the negative feedback signal in the closed loop control system. The mechanical strength of the anterior abdominal wall and abdominal capacity are significant factors determining feedback and satiety.

Keywords: Abdominal model; Capacity; Compliance; Dual sensing; Intraganglionic laminar endings; Intravenous nutritional infusion; LaPlace's law; Meal volume; Preloading; Satiety; Stiffness; Stomach model; Strain; Tension.

Satiety is the sensation of fullness that inhibits eating. The question is, how does the body sense satiety? This can be understood using an analogy to how an electronic scale senses weight. A scale has a rigid base that does not deform, which rests on a hard surface, the floor and a platform where weight is placed. Inside the scale, the platform transfers weight to a cantilever that is attached to the base. Fig. 3.1. On the top and bottom surfaces of the cantilever, between the base and the platform attachments, strain

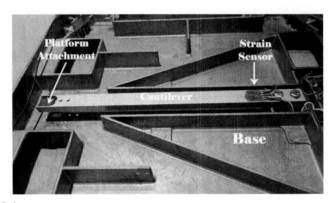

FIGURE 3.1

Electronic scale.

sensors are attached. Fig. 3.2 When weight is applied to the platform, mechanical force bends the soft metal of the cantilever, stretching the strain sensor on the top and compressing the strain sensor on the bottom. The cantilever bends from the force of the weight until the cantilever creates an equal and opposite force. When this is achieved no further bending occurs. Fig. 3.3. The strain sensor is a transducer which converts the mechanical weight to electrical energy, voltage. The conversion factor is voltage divided by pounds. Then, the voltage is transferred by wires to the central unit, which analyzes the signal and displays the weight. For a scale to accurately sense weight, the rigid base cannot deform with loading. If the base loses its mechanical strength and deforms, then less deformation occurs in the cantilever. Mechanical failure of the base results in inaccurate reduced weights.

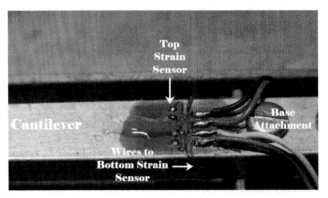

FIGURE 3.2

Strain sensors in an electronic scale.

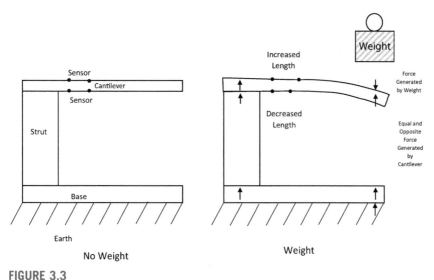

FIGURE 3.3

Cantilever deformation with weight loading.

Experiments in dogs have been performed to determine where in the gastrointestinal tract the satiety signal is generated. In one experiment, dogs underwent surgery to create a connection between the stomach and the external surface of the abdominal wall, a gastric fistula. After dogs ate, the food passed through the esophagus, entered the stomach, but then fell out of the stomach onto the floor. As a result of the fistula, the dogs would eat continuously until exhaustion, collapse, and upon reawakening repeat the cycle, never achieving satiety. From this the conclusion was drawn that food must be retained in the stomach or pass distally to achieve satiety.

The distal portion of the stomach has a valve called the pylorus. As the stomach is filled, small quantities of food are released by the valve, into the small intestine. Emptying the stomach can take several hours. On many occasions people eat meals quickly and achieve satiety after only a few minutes. Satiety is achieved while the majority of food is still within the stomach.[1] What property does food have prior to absorption?

Human studies have been performed, analyzing the meal volume eaten after nutritional preloading with either intragastric nutritional infusion or the caloric equivalent intravenous nutritional infusion.[2] The results show that intravenous nutritional infusion did not reduce the meal volume but intragastric nutritional volume preloading did. (This is the rational for serving soup as the first course in a meal.) Satiety is achieved by gastric volume sensation. The question is, how does the stomach sense volume?

The stomach is located in the left upper quadrant of the abdomen and has a capacity of 1—4 L in adults. The stomach is flexible and able to move within the abdominal cavity except at two points of attachment, proximately at the esophagus and distally at the duodenum. Fig. 3.4. The stomach has three major divisions. The fundus is the upper portion closest to the esophagus. The corpus is the central large portion and the antrum is the distal stomach. The stomach has two curves: the lesser curvature and the greater curvature. Both curves have attachments of omentum which consist of fat and blood vessels. Vertically, the stomach lies above the transverse colon and its fatty epiploic appendages. The stomach contains air and buoyancy is created by the surrounding structures.

The stomach wall is composed of four layers. From inside out, they are mucosa, submucosa, muscularis, and serosa. The muscularis is composed of three layers of smooth muscle. From the inside out, they are oblique, circular, and longitudinal. If the stomach sensed only intragastric volume,

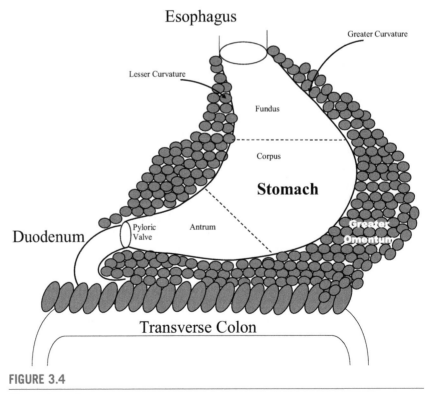

FIGURE 3.4

Stomach anatomy.

then the sensory cells should be located on the internal surface of the stomach. If the stomach sensed only extragastric volume, then the sensory cells should be located on the external surface of the stomach. However, neuroanatomic studies have shown two morphologically distinct types of sensory cells that are located within the muscular layers.[3] Intramuscular array are located within the muscle layers, run parallel to the muscle, and are believed to be length or stretch receptors. They are densely located in the fundus, moderate density in the corpus, but almost absent in the atrium. Intraganglionic laminar endings (IGLEs) are located between the circular and the longitudinal layers and are believed to be tension receptors.[3] They are most numerous in the antrum and corpus but absent in the fundus. Traditional electrophysiological testing of mechanical receptors have used internal distention as the stimulus. However, blunt tipped glass rods, gently touching the external surface of the stomach, are known to generate an electrical response. The IGLE cells may function as the biological equivalent of the strain sensor of an electronic scale and sense tension between the internal and external surfaces of the stomach. The IGLE cells are predominantly located in the distal stomach where food gravitates, before passing though the pylorus.

Engineering modeling techniques will be used to determine the forces acting upon the gastric sensory cells. The stomach is modeled as a flexible spheroid container of ingested food. The abdomen is modeled as a box with a rigid posterior wall (spine and ribs), side walls (ribs and iliac crest), and inferior floor (pelvis). Fig. 3.5. The top of the box is the flexible diaphragm that varies up and down from an average position. The anterior abdominal wall is elastic and consists of skin, fat, fascia, and muscle. Muscles are contained within the firm envelope of connective tissue called fascia. When a person sucks in their abdomen, the muscles flatten the abdominal wall. When the muscles relax, the fascia determines anterior projection. The anterior abdominal wall functions as the biological equivalent of the rigid base of an electrical scale that generates tension on the IGLE cells. The abdominal box contains fixed volume organs such as liver, spleen, kidneys, and pancreas. Rapid volume changes (minutes) occur from food ingestion. Slow volume changes (hours) result from intra-abdominal fat.

When volume is added to the box, the rigid surfaces cannot be displaced. The roof of the box is the last to displace because of the gravitational force on the abdominal contents. However, if diaphragmatic elevation did occur, it compromises respiration, which is immediately perceived and terminates additional volume increases. Compromised pulmonary function is

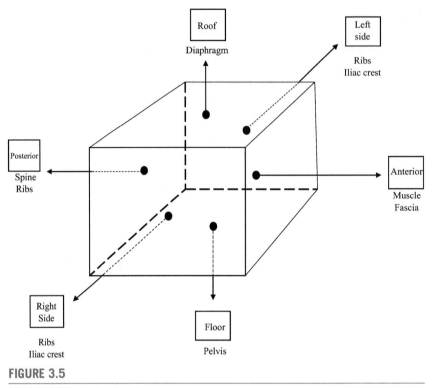

FIGURE 3.5

Model of the abdominal box.

a secondary system (fail-safe) that prevents meal volume overload. On Thanksgiving Day, people frequently overeat and present to the emergency room complaining of difficulty breathing. However, increased volume can force the elastic anterior abdominal wall to displace anteriorly. Anterior displacement is opposed by the mechanical strength of the fascia and muscle of the anterior abdominal wall. The stiffer the anterior abdominal wall, the less anterior displacement will occur. Compliance is the reciprocal of stiffness.

There is a complex mathematical relationship between volume and pressure within the abdomen. As volume is added to an elastic closed container, the pressure gradually increases, similar to hydrostatic pressure, until the container reaches capacity. Additional volume requires greater pressure to distend the elastic container. Fig. 3.6.

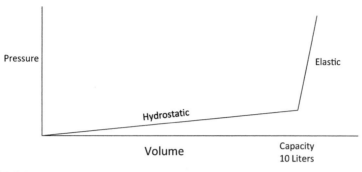

FIGURE 3.6

Pressure volume curve of the abdominal box.

The abdominal box is an elastic closed container and the intra-abdominal volume determines intra-abdominal pressure, depending on its capacity and compliance. Consider the two examples described in Fig. 3.7.

Example 1 is a small capacity abdomen that has a very stiff anterior abdominal wall (low compliance). This is analogous to a normal weight person with an elliptical transverse abdominal wall cross section and mechanically strong anterior abdominal wall. Example 2 is a large capacity abdomen and has a weak anterior abdominal wall (high compliance). This is analogous to an obese person with a round transverse abdominal cross section with a weak anterior abdominal wall. (These analogies will be discussed in greater detail in later chapters.) Increased capacity shifts the pressure volume curve to the right.

Compliance is mathematically defined as the change in volume divided by the change in pressure. $C = \Delta V/\Delta P$. The slope in the pressure volume curve is the reciprocal of compliance. Slope $= 1/C = \Delta P/\Delta V$. To achieve

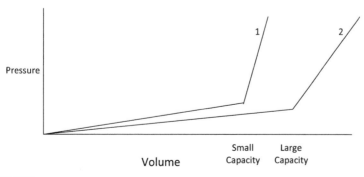

FIGURE 3.7

Pressure volume curve 1 is small capacity with stiff anterior abdominal wall and curve 2 is large capacity with weak anterior abdominal wall.

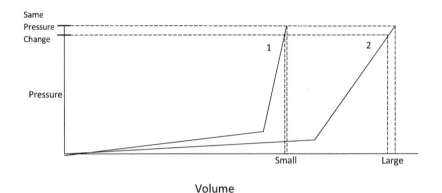

FIGURE 3.8

Pressure volume curve showing weak abdominal wall (2) requires larger volumes to achieve the same pressure change as the stiff abdominal wall (1).

the same change in pressure, a small volume is required for example 1, but a large volume is required for example 2. Fig. 3.8. Abdominal volume capacity is about 10 L and meal volume represents only a small portion of the total volume. We are not interested in the entire volume pressure curve but only the small portion that changes with meals. Fig. 3.9 is an enlargement of Fig. 3.8 focusing on changes associated with meals.

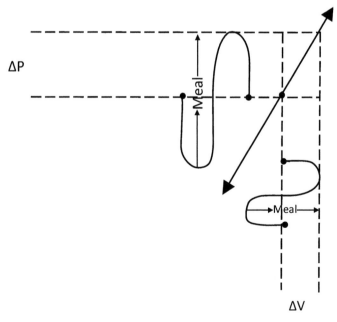

FIGURE 3.9

Meal volume pressure change Δ V, produces change Δ P, depending on the slope of the volume pressure curve.

The pressure volume curve in Fig. 3.9 can be approximated by a linear equation using the standard of mathematical formula of $Y = mX + b$. In this model, Y is pressure, X is volume, m is the slope $\Delta P/\Delta V$, which is $1/C$, and b is the Y axis intersect ($X = 0$) shown in Fig. 3.10. It is important to note that b is a negative number. The X axis intersect is determined by the equation $P = V/C + b$ when $P = 0$, therefore, $V = -bC$. Since b is negative, then V is positive. In this model, we will define $-bC$ as the capacity of the system. Pressure becomes positive after capacity is reached and this is the portion of the curve related to meals.

Consider what happens when a child grows into an adult and the abdominal box increases in capacity. Fig. 3.11 represents the pressure volume curve for a child, adolescent, and adult with the same compliance.

The value of b changes as shown in Fig. 3.11. Since b is a negative number, we will compare the absolute values of b. A child has a small capacity of the abdominal box and has a small absolute value of b. An adult

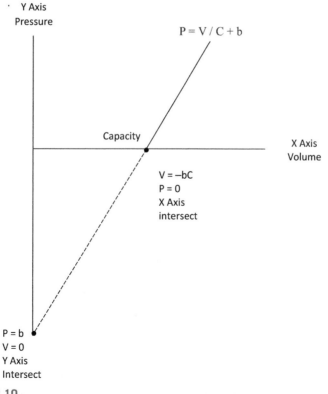

FIGURE 3.10

Linear approximation of the pressure volume curve that is valid over the volume domain related to meals.

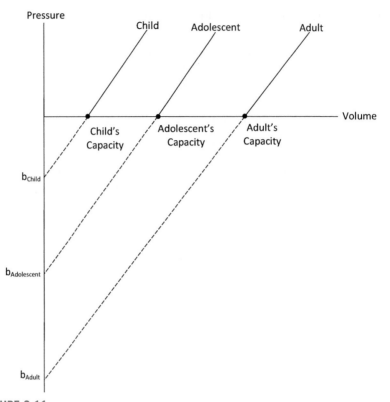

FIGURE 3.11

Linear approximation of the pressure volume curves for growth from childhood to adult.

has a large capacity of the abdominal box and has a large absolute value of b. As a child grows into an adult, growth hormone increases the bone length which increases the physical dimensions of the abdominal box and increases its capacity. The linear equations that describe the pressure volume curve, over the volume domain that corresponds to the meal volume is, $P = V/C + b$. The value of b is negative and its absolute value increases with increased abdominal box capacity. This equation will be used in Chapter 6 to explain why fat weight increases as children grow to become adults.

There is a different mathematical relationship between pressure and volume within the stomach. In this model, the stomach is not within the abdominal box. The stomach has the capacity to hold 1−4 L, but the meal volume normally does not extend to capacity and the elastic portion of the curve. Fig. 3.12.

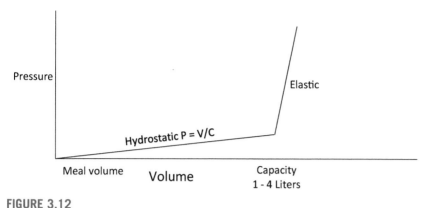

FIGURE 3.12

Pressure volume curve for the stomach.

In the hydrostatic region of the stomach's pressure volume curve, the slope m is $\Delta P/\Delta V = P/V = 1/C$. The Y axis intercept is 0, therefore $b = 0$. The standard mathematical form $Y = mX + b$ becomes $P = V/C$ and is valid within the domain of normal sized meals. In the treatment of obesity, bariatric surgeons often perform gastric restrictive procedures to decrease the capacity of the stomach. (These will be discussed in detail in later chapters.) Gastric operations shift the pressure volume curve to the left and reduce the stomach's capacity from 1 to 4 L down to 50−150 cm^3, depending on the procedure. The high compliance of the hydrostatic region has been replaced by the low compliance of the elastic region. This is done to increase the pressure within the stomach to terminate meals after ingestion of small volumes. The pressure volume relationship after restrictive bariatric surgery is $P = V_S/C_S + b_S$. Fig. 3.13. These changes in capacity and compliance are exactly the opposite of the changes in the anterior abdominal wall and abdominal box that occurred with obesity.

The volume pressure linear equations for the abdominal box and the stomach spheroid are combined to explain mathematically how meal volume creates satiety. Fig. 3.14. However, in this model, the stomach is within the abdominal box. Since the stomach is flexible, the intragastric pressure is equal to the intra-abdominal pressure plus the gastric wall pressure. The pressure volume curve for the stomach begins at the pressure and volume in the abdomen before meals. Fig. 3.15. Meal volume within the stomach creates small increases in pressure since the pressure volume curve functions in the hydrostatic region within capacity and with a high compliance. However, the same low volume added to the abdominal box creates a large increase in pressure since the pressure volume curve functions in the elastic region beyond capacity within a low compliance box.

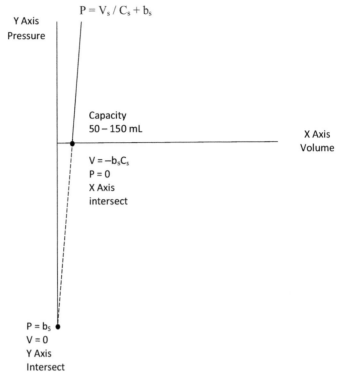

FIGURE 3.13

Pressure volume curve for the stomach after restrictive bariatric surgery reduces capacity to $50 - 150$ mL.

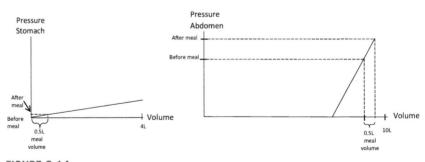

FIGURE 3.14

Pressure volume curve on the left displays a small increase in stomach pressure after 0.5 liter meal. Pressure volume curve on the right displays a large increase in intra-abdominal pressure after a 0.5 liter meal.

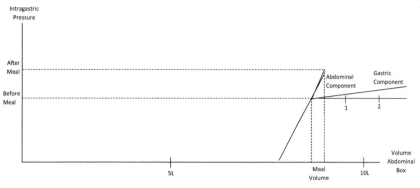

FIGURE 3.15

The pressure volume curve from combining the right and left pressure volume curves from figure 3.14. The change in intragastric pressure is the sum of the small intra-gastric increase in pressure and the large intra-abdominal increase in pressure.

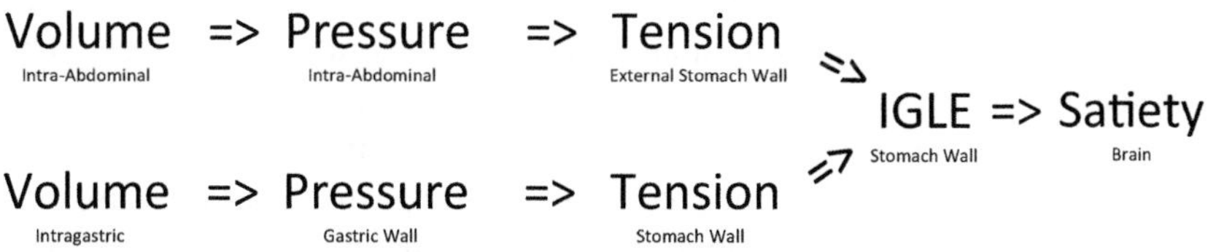

Volume => Pressure => Tension
Intra-Abdominal   Intra-Abdominal   External Stomach Wall

IGLE => Satiety
Stomach Wall   Brain

Volume => Pressure => Tension
Intragastric   Gastric Wall   Stomach Wall

FIGURE 3.16

IGLE sensors within the stomach wall create satiety by the combination of intra-abdominal volume and intra-gastric volume.

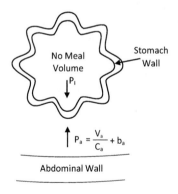

$$P_s = \frac{V_s}{C_s} + b_s$$

$$P_a = \frac{V_a}{C_a} + b_a$$

Abdominal Wall

Before A Meal

Intra-gastric pressure P_I is equal to Intra-abdominal pressure P_a.

After a Meal

Meal volume stretches the stomach wall and the stomach wall generates pressure P_s. Meal volume stretches the anterior abdominal wall and P_a increases until pressure is balanced.

$$P_I = P_a + P_s$$

FIGURE 3.17

Meal volume creates stomach wall pressure P_s and increases intra-abdominal pressure P_a. P_I is the sum of $P_s + P_s$ and increases with meals.

Fig. 3.16 shows the two components that create satiety. The equations are in Appendix 3.1 and are explained below.

Meal volume causes the internal stomach wall to expand and the external stomach wall to contract. Fig. 3.17. The intra-abdominal pressure P_a generated is equal to the intra-abdominal volume V_a divided by C_a plus b_a. Eq. (3.1) The gastric wall pressure P_s generated is equal to the gastric volume V_s divided by C_s plus b_s Eq. (3.2) Since the stomach wall is flexible, the wall deflects until the intragastric pressure P_I equals the sum of gastric wall pressure P_s and intra-abdominal pressure P_a. Eq. (3.3). As seen in Fig. 3.15, the greater pressure is determined by the abdominal box. However, with mechanical failure of the abdominal wall (increased capacity and increased compliance) or restrictive bariatric surgery this may not be true. These equations allow both pressure sources to be included; however, usually the abdominal wall pressure dominates. LaPlace's law states that tension equals pressure times radius. Eq. (3.4). The stomach is spheroid and each point on the surface has two radii. The intra-gastric pressure creates tension that expands the internal surface of the stomach. Fig. 3.18 Intra-abdominal pressure and gastric wall pressure creates tension in the IGLE sensors within the stomach wall. Fig. 3.19. The IGLE cells are dual sensing and they generate an electrical signal from the combination of gastric volume and intra-abdominal volume. The electrical signal is transmitted by the vagus nerve to the brain. When the signal reaches the threshold level, satiety is achieved.

The neuromechanical system determines satiety and is analogous to the electromechanical scale that determines weight. Fig. 3.20. The IGLE senses tension similar to the strain sensor. In the scale, the strut directly connects the cantilever to the base. Pressure from the anterior abdominal wall to the stomach wall is transmitted intra-abdominally hydraulically, pneumatically, or by direct physical contact. Accurate weight

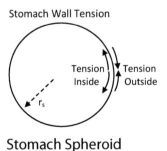

Stomach Wall Tension

Tension Inside   Tension Outside

r_s

Stomach Spheroid

FIGURE 3.18

The stomach is molded as a spheroid. Tension generated on the outside surface and inside surface is dependent on the radius of the stomach R_s and the pressure.

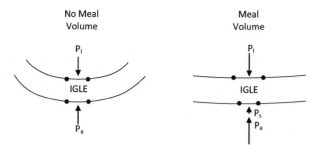

No Meal
Volume

P_I

IGLE

P_a

Points on the IGLE

Meal
Volume

P_I

IGLE

P_s
P_a

Points on the IGLE

Points near to the internal
surface will stretch by intragastric pressure P_I. Points near
to the external surface will
become closer by gastric wall
pressure P_s and intra-
abdominal pressure P_a.

FIGURE 3.19

IGLE tension sensors deform from meal volume.

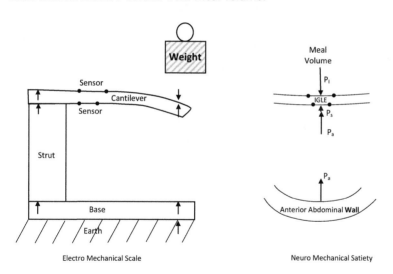

Electro Mechanical Scale

Neuro Mechanical Satiety

Comparison of Electro Mechanical Scale and Neuro Mechanical Satiety

Force	<=>	Meal volume
Strain Sensor	<=>	IGLE
Cantilever	<=>	Stomach Wall
Strut	<=>	Hydraulic, Pneumatic, Physical
Base	<=>	Anterior Abdominal Wall

FIGURE 3.20

Comparison of electro mechanical scale and neuro mechanical satiety.

requires a rigid base that does not deform. The anterior abdominal wall is the base for the neuromechanical system and rigidity is required for accurately determining satiety. Decreased mechanical strength of the anterior abdominal wall requires additional meal volume to achieve satiety.

Are there clinical studies that support the concept that anterior abdominal wall capacity and compliance are significant factors that determine meal volume, satiety, and weight?

Appendix 3.1

$$P_a = \frac{V_a}{C_a} + b_a \qquad\qquad 3.1$$

$$P_s = \frac{V_s}{C_s} + b_s \qquad\qquad 3.2$$

$$P_I = P_a + P_s \qquad\qquad 3.3$$

$$T = P_I \times r_s \qquad\qquad 3.4$$

$$T = (P_a + P_s)r_s \qquad\qquad 3.5$$

$$T = \frac{V_a r_s}{C_a} + b_a r_s + \frac{V_s r_s}{C_s} + b_s r_s \qquad\qquad 3.6$$

$$\text{Definition } S_a = \frac{r_s}{C_a} \qquad\qquad 3.7$$

$$\text{Definition } S_s = \frac{r_s}{C_s} \qquad\qquad 3.8$$

$$T = V_a S_a + b_a r_s + V_s S_s + b_s r_s \qquad\qquad 3.9$$

References

1. Deutsch J. Signal determining meal size. In: *Eating Habits.* John Wiley & Sons Ltd.; 1987:155−173.
2. Shide D, et al. Accurate energy compensation for intragastric and oral nutrients in lean males. *Am J Clin Nutr.* 1995;61:754−764.
3. Phillips R, Powely T. Tension and stretch receptors on gastrointestinal smooth muscle: Re-evaluating vagal mechanorecepter electrophysiology. *Brain Res Rev.* 2000;34:1−26.

Serendipity

Abstract

After pregnancy, women frequently want the restore their prepregnancy figure. This usually requires an abdominoplasty. Abdominoplasties excise excess skin and repair the internal support layer called fascia. While performing abdominoplasties, I noted the facial layer was frequently damaged and sutures failed to hold. I began using an overlay of artificial material called mesh to reinforce the repair. The mesh decreases the volume of the abdominal cavity and increases the mechanical strength of the abdominal wall directly and indirectly by shortening the stretched muscle of the abdominal wall (Starling's law). Afterward, women experience increased work of breathing and stated that they were not hungry for several days, ate smaller meals, and lost weight. From these observations, I concluded that the mechanical strength of the anterior abdominal wall is a major determent of meal volume, satiety, and weight.

Keywords: Elastic modulus; Fascia; Hernia; Mesh; Mommy makeover; Muscle; Starling's law; Work of breathing.

During my first week in medical school, a professor spoke of the importance of clinical observation. He told the story of a rheumatologist in Illinois who had treated his arthritic patients with aspirin. After many years in practice, the rheumatologist noted that none of his patients had myocardial infarctions (heart attacks). From this clinical observation, the therapeutic value of aspirin in the prevention of heart disease was established.

As a plastic surgeon, I frequently consult women who want their prepregnancy figure restored. The "mommy makeover" has several components including tummy tucks. After pregnancy, the abdominal wall requires surgery in three anatomical layers: skin, fat, and fascia. The skin is composed of two layers: the epidermis and dermis. The epidermis is the outer layer that regulates water loss and prevents infection. The dermis is the inner layer that provides mechanical strength and elastic recoil. During pregnancy, the expanded uterus stretches the skin and stretch marks are visible tears in the dermis from expansion beyond the elastic modulus of the dermis. Tummy tucks require excision of excess skin and redraping the remaining skin to close the wound. Weight gain during pregnancy results in increased fat storage within the abdominal wall which is resected simultaneous with the skin resection. The fascia layer, like the dermis, undergoes stretching by the expanding uterus and tears, due to expansion beyond its elastic modulus. Unlike stretch marks, fascial tears can only be seen intraoperatively (Fig. 4.1). There are multiple layers of fascia but only the outer layer is visible. To restore an hourglass figure, the fascia must be tightened. Fascial sutures are placed horizontally on both sides of the midline from the sternum to the pubic bone, pulling the fascia horizontally toward the midline. During my first few years in private practice, I preformed the traditional skin and fat resection with fascial tightening. During surgery, I observed that after I sutured the fascia in the midline, the remaining fascia stretched, separated, or tore. I then used additional sutures, to repair these defects.

While in undergraduate school studying electrical engineering, one of my professors, Wen H. Ko, told the class, when designing a circuit "design right first time, no patch, patch, patch." I think of plastic surgery as human engineering and I applied his principals to my tummy tucks. Instead of multiple patches in the fascia, I decided to use a large piece of mesh to reinforce the fascia of the inferior portion of the anterior abdominal

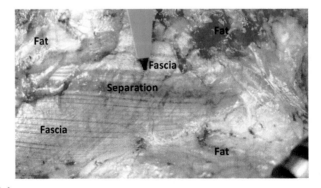

FIGURE 4.1

Fascial separation after pregnancy.

wall, which bears the greatest mechanical load. Mesh has been used since the 1950s for hernia repair. Hernias are complete tears of all the layers of the fascia and muscle, that allow intraabdominal contents to displace outward to the under surface of the skin. Since mesh is therapeutic for complete tears that occur in hernias, it is effective for stretching, separation or partial tears after pregnancy. Mesh increases the mechanical strength of the anterior abdominal wall directly by the physical strength of the mesh and indirectly by Starling's law (Fig. 4.2). Starling's law states that muscle strength is greatest at normal length. When the overstretched muscle after pregnancy is shortened, toward its normal length by applying mesh, the muscle's mechanical strength increases.

I began using mesh routinely on all women who did not desire future pregnancies since it does not stretch (Fig. 4.3). Postoperatively, the women were not hungry, did not eat for several days, and experienced increased work breathing. After several days, the breathing returned to normal, patients experienced early satiety and ate less than preoperatively. They also reported weight loss of amounts significantly greater than the amount removed at surgery. We published an article describing our results of Abdominoplasty With Mesh Reinforcement, in Plastic and Reconstructive Surgery, September 2011—Volume 126-Issue 3-p149e-150e. This was a 3-year retrospective review that analyzed the results of mesh reinforcement in two groups. The first had only anterior rectus sheath

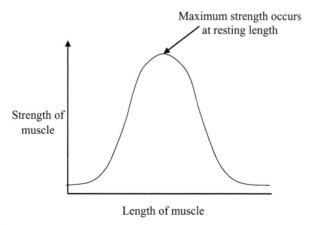

FIGURE 4.2

Starling's law.

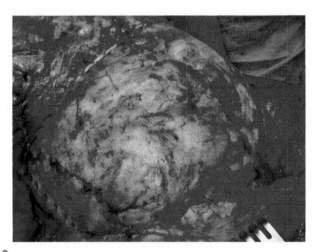

FIGURE 4.3

Abdominoplasty with mesh reinforcement.

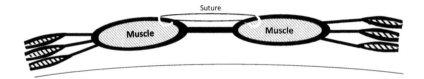

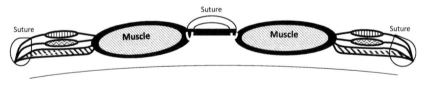

FIGURE 4.4

Horizontal cross sections of the anterior abdominal wall. Top figure shows anterior rectus sheath plication. Bottom figure shows linear alba plication and bilateral lateral plications.

plication, and the second group had bilateral lateral plications plus plication of the linea alba (Fig. 4.4). Both groups had mesh applied over the fascial repairs. In the first group, 33% had weight loss at 36 months. In the second group, 86% had weight loss at 36 months. The second group was subdivided in to four groups based on body mass index. The body mass index reduction for each subgroup was 0.4, 1.9, 3.5, and 5.3 kg/m^2 for the normal weight, overweight, obese, and extremely obese, respectively. These findings suggest that the second abdominoplasty group with mesh reinforcement specifically corrects the pathology associated with increased weight. The abdominal capacity was decreased by the triple plication and the compliance decreased by the mesh. The compliance of the anterior abdominal wall and the abdominal capacity are significant components determining meal volume, satiety, and weight.

The neuromechanical hypothesis

Chapter outline

Abstract

The neuromechanical hypothesis states that weight is regulated by a neuromechanical dual closed loop control system. Eating begins the fast loop cycle, which increases intragastric volume and intra-abdominal volume. Tension in the stomach wall causes the IGLE tension receptors to transmit an electrical signal through the vagus nerve to the nuclease tractus solitaruis and the hypothalamic satiety center. When this signal exceeds the internal reference volume, satiety is achieved, and eating is terminated. Meal volume is switched by the pylorus into the intestines, beginning the slow loop cycle. If energy demands during the slow cycle exceed the caloric intake, then stored fat is consumed which decreases intra-abdominal volume. When eating resumes, then meal volume will increase to compensate. If energy demands during the slow cycle are less than the caloric intake, then excess fat will be stored, which increases intra-abdominal volume. When eating resumes, meal volume will decrease to compensate.

Keywords: Conversation factor K; Fast cycle; Fat volume equation; Hypothalamus; Intra-abdominal nonfat volume; Meal volume equation; Neuromechanical dual closed loop; Nucleus tractus solitaruis; Pyloric switch; Satiety equation; Scientific method; Slow cycle; Theory of weight regulation.

Weight Regulation and Curing Acquired Obesity. https://doi.org/10.1016/B978-0-323-77854-1.00005-6
39

Scientific method is a procedure that requires a series of steps. An observation is made, a question is generated, a hypothesis is formulated, an experiment is performed, the data are analyzed, and a conclusion is drawn. The observation was that abdominoplasty with mesh reinforcement achieved satiety with less meal volume which resulted in weight loss. The question is, how is weight regulated? Currently, there are no proven theories of weight regulation.

The hypothesis is that weight is regulated by a neuromechanical dual closed loop control system. Fig. 5.1. The fast cycle occurs within minutes and originates from meal volume within the stomach, which increases intragastric pressure and meal volume within the intra-abdominal compartment, which increases intra-abdominal pressure. The intra-abdominal fat volume at the beginning of the meal does not change during the fast cycle because the meal is within the stomach. Fig. 5.2. Intragastric pressure equals gastric wall pressure plus intra-abdominal pressure and produces gastric wall tension by LaPlace's law. The IGLE tension receptors within the intramuscular layers of the stomach sense gastric wall and intra-abdominal pressure which generates a signal. This is analogous to the electrical signal generated by the strain sensors in the electronic scale described in Chapter 3. The IGLE receptors convert tension to an electrical signal that represents volume. Volume equals wall tension times the conversion factor K. The IGLE signal is conducted by the vagus nerve to the nucleus tractus solitaries in the brain stem. Fig. 5.3. The nucleus tractus solitarius connects with the hypothalamus satiety center. Within the hypothalamus an internal volume reference signal is compared to the negative feedback volume signal. If the feedback signal is greater than the reference signal, satiety is achieved, and eating should terminate. If the feedback signal is less than the reference signal, satiety has not been achieved, hunger is perceived and eating continues. Fig. 5.4 The hypothalamus connects with the motor cortex to activate the peripheral motor nerves necessary to perform the physical act of eating. The satiety equation is derived from Fig. 5.2 and states that meal volume M is inversely related to total fat volume. Appendix 5.1. $M = C_1 - C_2 O$, where C_1 and C_2 are constant values determined by the parameters of the neuromechanical model. Meal volume is determined by fat volume at the beginning of the fast cycle.

The two cycles of the dual loop alternate. Satiety ends the fast cycle and begins the slow cycle. The meal volume is switched by the pylorus from the stomach to the intestines and the intragastric volume decreases to zero. The fat is absorbed by the intestines and distributed by the vascular system throughout the body as needed. The energy required to meet demands consumes some or all of the absorbed fat volume or may even require reabsorption of previously stored fat. After the energy demands are satisfied and the fat is redistributed, the intra-abdominal volume generates tension on the external surface of the gastric wall. The slow feedback control system is modeled in Fig. 5.5 and is used to derive the total fat volume equation. $O = [(R/KS_a) - N - b_aC_a]/D$ Appendix 5.2. Total fat volume is determined by the meal volume at the beginning of the slow cycle. For this system to regulate total fat volume (F dominant), the product $KS_aDA_AA_BA_C$ must be much greater than 1. When this condition is met, then the total fat volume O is dependent on the brain's internal volume reference R, distribution ratio D, nonfat intra-abdominal volume N, conversion factor K, and S_a. S_a determines the tension on the external surface of the stomach. The stiffer the anterior abdominal wall (lower compliance), the greater the tension on the external stomach wall. S_a equals radius of the stomach r_s divided by the compliance of the anterior abdominal wall C_a.

The neuromechanical dual closed loop control system differs significantly from electronic control systems. In an electronic control system, the input to output change is determined by the speed of light (3×10^{10} cm/s). If an electronic closed loop was approximately 3 cm long, then the output would change in 3 cm/3×10^{10} cm/s $= 10^{-10}$ s (0.1 nano second). The neuromechanical dual closed loop control system has two cycles that operate at two different rates. The fast cycle lasts approximately several minutes, and the slow cycle lasts several hours.

The neuromechanical model is valid when caloric intake is greater than or equal to caloric expenditure (positive or neutral caloric balance, respectively). When caloric intake is less than caloric expenditures (negative calorie balance), weight loss occurs at a rate of 1 pound per 3500 Kcal deficiency. Although we have focused on the neuromechanical components, weight regulation also requires biochemical reactions within the components.

The Neuromechanical Hypothesis Summary

1. Weight is regulated by a neuromechanical dual closed loop control system when positive or neutral caloric balance exists. Weight is reduced at 1 pound per 3500 kcals when negative caloric balance occurs.
2. The fast cycle compares the reference volume to the feedback volume and determines the meal volume. Meal volume is not constant but is inversely related fat volume to by equation $M = C_1 - C_2O$. Appendix 5.1. This loop functions as a high gain inverter (relative to O) and does not regulate meal volume.
3. The pylorus functions as a switch that transfers food from the stomach to the small intestines during the slow cycle. Intra-abdominal volume progressively decreases due to absorption and elimination of GI

contents, urination, and fat consumption. Eventually the satiety achieved during the fast cycle is lost and hunger returns. The slow cycle ends, and the fast cycle begins with eating.

4. When the product $KS_aDA_AA_BA_C$ is much, much greater than one, and the stiffness of the anterior abdominal wall is greater than the stiffness of the stomach wall, then fat volume is regulated in the slow cycle by the equation. Fig. 5.6.

$$O = \frac{(R/KS_a) - N - b_aC_a}{D}$$

5. S_a equals radius of the stomach r_s divided by compliance of the anterior abdominal wall C_a,

$$S_a = \frac{r_s}{C_a}$$

$$\text{Fat volume} \ \ O = \frac{(RC_a/Kr_s) - N - b_aC_a}{D}$$

6. Since b_a is negative, then $-b_aC_a$ is a positive number that is determined by the capacity of the intra-abdominal box. Increased capacity of the abdominal box $-b_aC_a$, R, and C_a increased fat volume O. K, r_s, D, and N decrease fat volume O.

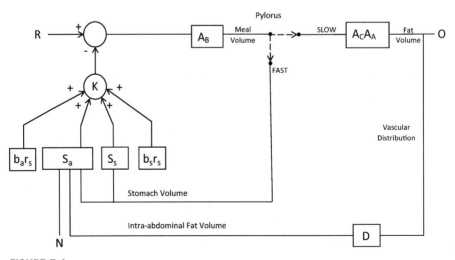

FIGURE 5.1

Neuro mechanical dual closed loop model.

Neuromechanical model

1. The dual loops consist of a fast cycle loop and a slow cycle loop.
2. Meal volume is switched by the pylorus from the stomach to the intestines.
3. S_s equals the radius of the stomach divided by the compliance of the stomach.
4. S_a equals the radius of the stomach divided by the compliance of anterior abdominal wall.
5. b_a is a negative number determined by the capacity of the abdominal box.
6. b_s is usually zero but may be a negative number after restrictive bariatric surgery.
7. r_s is radius of the stomach.
8. K is the conversion factor for tension to volume.

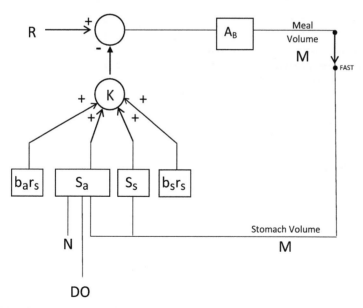

FIGURE 5.2

Fast cycle loop

Fast cycle loop

1. Meal volume M is completely within the stomach.
2. DO is a fixed value that represents intra-abdominal fat volume at the beginning of the meal.
3. N is a fixed value that represents intra-abdominal nonfat volume.
4. $S_a = r_s/C_a$ when r_s is the radius of the stomach and C_a is the compliance of the anterior abdominal wall.
5. b_a is a negative number determined by the capacity of the abdomen.
6. Fast satiety is achieved when the feedback volume is greater than the reference volume.

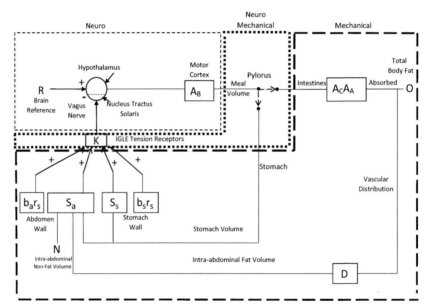

FIGURE 5.3

Neuro, neuromechanical and mechanical components of the model.

Neuromechanical model anatomy and physiology

1. The IGLE tension receptors are a mechanical to neuro transducer that converts tension to volume.
2. The motor cortex transmits through the peripheral nerves to the muscles required for eating which are neuro to mechanical transducers.
3. The pylorus is a neuromechanical switch.

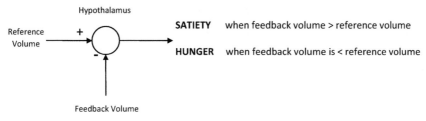

FIGURE 5.4

Hypothalamus determines hunger or satiety by comparing reference volume to feedback volume.

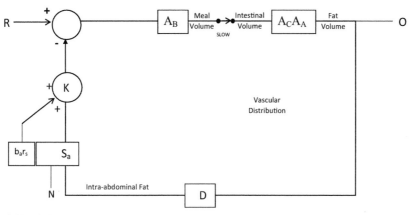

FIGURE 5.5

Slow cycle loop.

Slow closed loop

1. The stomach is empty, the fast loop has zero volume, and b_s is zero.
2. The meal volume is absorbed by the intestines and distributed in the slow closed loop.
3. N is nonfat intra-abdominal volume.
4. $b_a r_s$ is a negative number determined by of the radius of the stomach and the capacity of the abdominal box.
5. The satiety achieved in the fast cycle is maintained in the slow cycle until the feedback volume is less than the reference volume and hunger recurs.

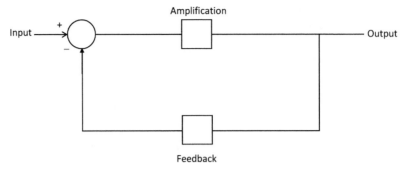

FIGURE 5.6

Neuro mechanical summary model.

Neuromechanical summary model

Input $= R - KS_aN - Kb_ar_s$
Amplification $= A_BA_CA_A$
Output $= O$
Feedback $= KDS_a$

This model assumes

1. The system is F dominant with $KS_aDA_AA_BA_C \gg 1$
2. $S_a \gg S_s$
3. $b_s =$ zero

Note:

1. b_a is a negative number, then $-b_ar_s$ is a positive number.
2. $R - KS_aN - Kb_ar_s$ can be considered as the reference.
3. The input values of K, S_a, N, r_s, and b_a are mathematically as important as R in determining the input and therefore the output of the control system.

Appendix 5.1

Satiety equation

Derived from Fig. 5.2

$$(R - KS_aDO - KS_aN - KS_aM - b_ar_s - b_sr_s - KS_sM)A_B = M$$

$$RA_B - KS_aDOA_B - KS_aNA_B - KS_aMA_B - b_ar_sA_B - b_sr_sA_B$$
$$-KS_sMA_B = M$$

$$RA_B - KS_aDOA_B - KS_aNA_B - b_ar_sA_B - b_sr_sA_B$$
$$= M(1 + KS_aA_B + KS_sA_B)$$

$$\frac{RA_B - KS_aNA_B - b_ar_sA_B - b_sr_sA_B}{1 + KS_aA_B + KS_sA_B} - \frac{KS_aDA_BO}{1 + KS_aA_B + KS_sA_B} = M$$

Simplified to

$$C_1 - C_2O = M$$

where

$$C_1 = \frac{RA_B - KS_aNA_B - b_ar_sA_B - b_sr_sA_B}{1 + KS_aA_B + KS_sA_B}$$

$$C_2 = \frac{KS_aDA_B}{1 + KS_aA_B + KS_sAB}$$

These are the correct values for all conditions.

Assuming the stiffness of the anterior abdominal wall is much greater than the stiffness of the stomach wall $(S_a \gg S_s)$, therefore, $KS_aA_B \gg KS_sA_B$ and KS_sA_B can be discarded. For the system to be F dominant, then $KS_aA_B \gg 1$, therefore 1 is also discarded, then

$$C_1 = \frac{R - b_ar_s - b_sr_sNKS_a}{ks_a} \qquad C_2 = \frac{DKS_a}{KS_a}$$

Therefore,

$$\frac{R - KS_aN - b_ar_s - b_sr_s - KS_aDO}{KS_a} = M$$

Reduced to

$$\frac{R - b_ar_s - b_sr_s}{KS_a} - N - DO = M$$

When b_s is zero for normal stomachs that have not had restrictive bariatric surgery,

Satiety equation is

$$\frac{R - b_ar_s}{KS_a} - N - DO = M$$

Meal volume M is inversely related to total fat volume O.

Appendix 5.2
Fat volume equation

Derived from Fig. 5.5

$$[R - Kb_a r_s - KS_a(N + DO)]A_B A_C A_A = O$$

$$(R - Kb_a r_s - KS_a N - KS_a DO)A_B A_C A_A = O$$

$$RA_A A_B A_C - Kb_a r_s A_A A_B A_C - KS_a N A_B A_C A_A - KS_a DO A_A A_B A_C = O$$

$$RA_A A_B A_C - Kb_a r_s A_A A_B A_C - KS_a N A_A A_B A_C = O(1 + KS_a DA_A A_B A_C)$$

$$\frac{RA_A A_B A_C - Kb_a r_s A_A A_B A_C - KS_a N A_A A_B A_C}{1 + KS_a DA_A A_B A_C} = O$$

These are the correct values for all conditions.

For the system to be F dominant, then $KS_a DA_A A_B A_C \gg 1$, therefore 1 is discarded, then

$$\frac{R/KS_a - b_a r_s/S_a - N}{D}$$

where

$$S_a = \frac{\text{Radius of Stomach}}{\text{Compliance of Abdominal wall}} = \frac{r_s}{C_a}$$

$$\text{fat volume equation } O = \frac{RC_a/Kr_s - b_a C_a - N}{D}$$

When $KS_a DA_A A_B A_C$ is much greater than 1 (F dominant), then the total fat volume depends on the reference R, nonfat intra-abdominal volume N, distribution ratio D, conversion factor K, and compliance of the abdominal wall C_a, radius of the stomach r_s, and $-b_a C_a$ which is the capacity of the abdominal box.

Animal experiments and human studies

6

Chapter outline

Abstract

A hypothesis must be consistent with previous observations. In Plication of Abdominoplasties with Marlex Mesh, Marquet showed that mesh reduced eating and weight. Carlson published a study on hysterectomy, showing weight increased after removal of intra-abdominal masses. Gastric sleeves decrease the compliance of the stomach, increase the radius, which increases the tension on the IGLE sensors, resulting in weight loss. Liposuction reduces extra-abdominal fat which increases the distribution ratio and the feedback, producing permanent weight reduction. All of these human studies are supportive of the hypothesis. Multiple animal experiments were also reviewed including Koopman's article on One-Way Crossed Intestine Transfer in Parabiotic Rats. This complex study disproved the humeral mechanism of satiety and proved an inverse relationship between meal volume and fat volume. His results are identical to the meal volume equation predicted by the hypothesis. Dark's study on the circannual cycle of squirrels supports the concept of an internal reference.

Keywords: Animal experiments; Circannual cycle; Fat index; Gastric banding; Gastric sleeve; Human studies; Hysterectomy; Leiomyoma; Liposuction; Literature search; Meal index; Meal volume equation; One-way crossed intestines; Parabiosis.

After the hypothesis is formulated, the next step is to design an experiment. Unfortunately, as a solo plastic surgeon, in a private practice, I did not have the facilities nor the funding necessary to perform animal experiments or conduct human studies. Instead, we began a search of the medical literature. The coauthor, Elisa Gonzalez, obtained her Physician Assistant degree from the University of Texas Medical Branch at Galveston, which gave us access to the Moody Medical Library.

We first searched the plastic surgical literature to see if other physicians had observed weight loss after abdominoplasty with mesh reinforcement. We discovered an article in the Annals of Plastic Surgery, published in 1995, by Marquet et al. from Brazil.[1] They described weight loss in 14 of 18 women (78%) after abdominoplasty with mesh reinforcement. Although their study contained less patients than ours, had shorter follow-up (mean of 19 months), and was not stratified by BMI, it did support our hypothesis. Marked decrease eating was their explanation for weight loss. The human studies of Marquet et al. and ours have shown that mesh reinforcement decreases weight. The mesh increases the mechanical strength of the anterior abdominal wall which decreases the compliance and plication reduces the abdominal capacity. These studies support the neuromechanical hypothesis and the fat volume equation $O = [(RC_a/Kr_s) - b_aC_a - N]/D$.

Further literature search revealed no other articles involving abdominoplasty with mesh reinforcement and weight regulation. Our search of human studies was expanded to include control system theory, weight, and satiety. Since our hypothesis has never been presented, we were unable to find any articles that proved or disproved it. It was our opinion that with the large volume of research devoted to obesity, there had to be pertinent human studies or animal experiments.

Eventually, we came upon a series of articles by Henry S. Koopman, involving control systems and satiety.[2] Internal Signals Cause Large Changes In Food Intake In One-Way Crossed Intestinal Rats was published in Brain Research Bulletin, Volume 14 Page 595−603 in 1985. This article is essential reading for anyone interested in weight regulation. In this study, 15 pairs of inbred males Lewis rats were sewn together, side to side over the abdominal wall. Fig. 6.1. The parabiosis created vascular anastomosis (connections) with 1% of the rat's blood exchanged per minute. After 3 hours, there was complete mixing of the blood. The blood exchange assured that any blood-borne hormone or unknown factor would rapidly equilibrate in both animals.

A second operation was performed that transected the midduodenum (upper small intestine) in both rats of the pair. In one rat of the pair, the recipient, a second transection was performed 30 cm distal in the intestine. This isolated, 30-centimeter segment was transferred into the other, donor rat and interposed between the two ends of the transected duodenum. The recipient rat had the two ends of the 30-centimeter gap brought together and closed. This was done for six pairs of rats. Another six pairs of rats

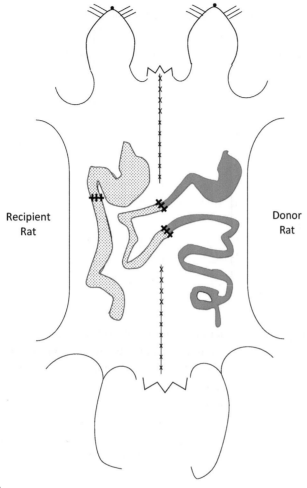

FIGURE 6.1

Koopman's one way crossed intestinal transfer. A portion of the recipient rats (red) small intestines are interposed into the donor rats (green) gastrointestinal tract.

had the same procedure except that only 15 cm were transferred. The remaining three pairs of rats had one or two intestinal transections with direct repairs (sham operations) without transfers and served as controls. After 24 hours, to allow intestinal healing, the rats were allowed to eat ad lib for 2–3 months during the study. At sacrifice the skin, carcass, fat, liver, heart, kidney, intestine, testis, and total weight were recorded for all five groups. Table 6.1 is derived from Koopman's original data and displays the total weight, meal volume, and total fat volume for the 30 cm donors, 15 cm donors, controls, 15 cm recipients, and 30 cm recipients.

Table 6.1 Koopman's original data converted to total fat volume.

	30 cm donor (%)	15 cm donor (%)	Control (%)	15 cm recipient (%)	30 cm recipient (%)
Animal weight grams	332 ± 9	352 ± 9	441 ± 15	416 ± 12	413 ± 11
Meal volume for 24 h cm³	128 ± 11	102 ± 17	76 ± 22	65 ± 11	52 ± 43
Total fat weight grams	17 ± 23	21 ± 13	41 ± 31	44 ± 15	47 ± 26
Total fat volume cm³	19 ± 23	23 ± 13	46 ± 31	49 ± 15	52 ± 26

All the groups were genetically identical and allowed to eat to satiety. There was an inverse relationship between meal volume and total fat volume. Fig. 6.2. From his data, the equation, meal volume = 160−2.1 fat volume is derived. If satiety was achieved by food volume in the stomach alone, then the rats should have eaten the same volume. If the satiety signal was transmitted to the brain by blood-borne factors, then the meal volume should be the same. This study proves that food in the stomach alone does not create satiety. In the summary of Dr. Koopman's article he states, "Signals from the lower small intestine and from the body fat may also play a role in the long-term change in feeding behavior." After reading his articles, I called Dr. Koopman and spoke to him on two occasions. At the first, we discussed the fact that all the rats gained weight during the study. He explained that young, growing rats were used. The importance of this is that with positive caloric balance, the weight control system would be adding weight for all five groups. The neuromechanical hypothesis is only valid for positive or neutral caloric balance; therefore, it is valid for this animal model. At the second call, I discussed my concepts of weight regulation. At the end of that call, Dr. Koopman told me he no longer believed that the small intestine was a determining factor in weight regulation. I agreed and told him that I believe weight regulation is controlled by the stomach.

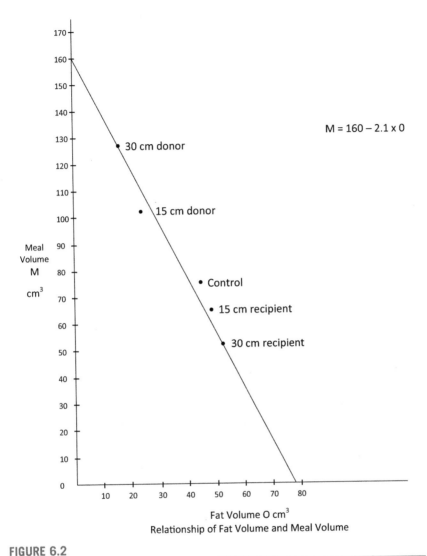

$M = 160 - 2.1 \times 0$

FIGURE 6.2

Relationship of fat volume and meal volume fat volume O cm^3.

Dr. Koopman's data can be interpreted in an alternate way. Consider the control rat as normal with a normal fat volume and consumes a normal meal volume. The donor and recipient rats have abnormal lower or higher fat volumes, respectively. The fat volumes and meal volumes are compared to the normal fat volume and normal meal volume, respectively. The fat index equals fat volume divided by control fat volume. The meal index equals meal volume divided by control meal volume. The fat index and meal index

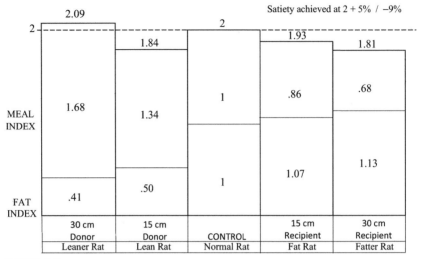

FIGURE 6.3

An alternate interpretation of Koopman's data showing that satiety is achieved when the meal index plus the fat index equals 2 + 5% / −9%.

for all five groups are shown in Fig. 6.3 and were derived from Table 6.1. The normal rats had 1 unit of fat and ate 1 unit meals to achieve satiety. The donor rats had an abnormally lower fat index and compensated by eating higher than normal meal index to achieve satiety. The recipient rats had an abnormally higher fat index and compensated by eating a lower meal index to achieve satiety. In summary, when rats have more than normal fat, they eat less than normal and when they have less fat than normal they eat more. In all rats, satiety was achieved when the rats ate a meal index that when combined with the fat index equals 2 + 5% / −9%. The intra-abdominal fat volume is determined by the fat distribution ratio, which is the same for all the inbred rats of the study. Fat and nonfat volume within the intra-abdominal box combined with the meal volume creates tension in the wall of the stomach resulting in satiety. Dr. Koopman's study supports the neuromechanical hypothesis with feedback occurring from the meal and intra-abdominal fat with the satiety signal transmitted to the brain by the vagus nerve. The equation meal volume = 160−2.1 fat volume is mathematically identical to the satiety equation $M = C_1 - C_2 O$. Dr. Koopman's study supports the fast loop of the hypothesis.

John Dark et al. published several studies on adipose tissue removal in female brown squirrels.[3] Squirrels have a circannual cycle with peak weight in fall and trough in spring. During the cycle, the fat changes, but no adipose tissue sites were underutilized or overutilized. The number of fat cells did not change but the fat volume per cell did change. Therefore, the distribution ratio is unchanged. In his experiments, 50%—85% of retroperitoneal and parametrial (both are intra-abdominal) fat and 50% —85% of inguinal subcutaneous (extra-abdominal) fat were removed. Irrespective of the phase of the circannual cycle, within 2 months of the fat removal, the squirrels restored body mass to the value appropriate to their circannual cycle. In their discussion, they state "Accurate compensation in body mass achieved after removal of a substantial portion of body fat suggests that feedback from the body lipid reserves is considerably precise. The mechanism involved in detecting a body mass defect after lipectomy and in an accurate compensation for the defect are presently unknown." That was stated in 1984.

As a plastic surgeon, I frequently perform liposuction and remove 5 L (10 lbs.) of extra-abdominal fat. After surgery, the patients have permanently decreased weight and do not compensate for fat reduction.[4] Table 6.2. Liposuction reduces extra-abdominal fat which increases the distribution ratio D. Intra-abdominal fat is unchanged, so there is no change in intra-abdominal volume. In the fat weight equation, increased D decreases total fat volume resulting in weight reduction. If total fat was sensed or the extra-abdominal fat that was removed was sensed, then compensation should occur. Compensation did not occur, therefore total fat is not sensed, nor is the fat removed by liposuction. This is consistent with the hypothesis that only intra-abdominal fat is sensed.

In the studies by Dark et al., both intra-abdominal and extra-abdominal fat was removed. The amount removed was 50%—85% in both, intra-abdominally and extra-abdominally, therefore the distribution ratio D did not change. However, since intra-abdominal fat was removed, and is sensed, the neuromechanical model predicts that meal volume will increase. The increased meal volume restored the intra-abdominal fat to the previous amount and simultaneously restored the extra-abdominal fat volume. The slow loop equation determines fat volume by $O = [(RC_a/Kr_s) - b_aC_a - N]/D$. Squirrels have a circannual cycle that corresponds to a changing R value in the equation. The value of D is unchanged and R changed during the 2 months required for the weight to return to the predetermined value in the circannual cycle. The fat volume equation is consistent with the observations of both the human liposuction study and Dark et al. animal experiments.

Table 6.2 Comparison of extra-abdominal only and combined intra-abdominal and extra-abdominal fat removal.

Fat removed	Total fat volume O	Intra-abdominal fat volume	Extra-abdominal fat volume	Distribution ratio $D\ \frac{I}{I+E}$	Removed fat sensed	Total fat equation predicts $O \propto \frac{1}{D}$	Observed change in total fat O	Reference R
Extra-abdominal human studies	↓	No change	↓	↑	No	↓	Permanent ↓	No change
Intra-abdominal + extra-abdominal animal experiments John Dark.et al.	↓	↓	↓	No change	Yes	No change	Returns to predicted in 2 months	Varies with season ↓↑

We know that fat volume increases as a child grows into an adult. One possible explanation would be that the value of R changes with age. Pediatric age, height, weight, and BMI tables[5] in the 50th percentile for boys age 2 to 16 show that BMI increases 21% (16.9−20.5), weight increases 376% (12.8−61 kg), length increases 100% (87−174 cm), and length squared increases 300%. If R changed during growth, then it must be synchronized with growth hormone, since the BMI is relatively constant and depends on length squared. Growth hormone controls bone length, which determines the capacity of the abdomen $-b_aC_a$. In the fat volume equation $O = [(RC_a/Kr_s) − N − b_aC_a]/D$, increased capacity results at increased fat volume. We do not need to invoke changes in R to explain fat volume increased with growth. Growth hormone alone may explain it, and the value of R may remain constant throughout a human's life.

N represents intra-abdominal nonfat volume. Any operation that removes nonfat intra-abdominal volume would be expected to increase total fat weight. Carlson et al. published a prospective study on hysterectomy with 1 year follow-up.[6] The most frequent indication for hysterectomy was leiomyoma in 35% of patients. Leiomyomas (fibroids) are a noncancerous muscle tumor of the uterus that can reach the size of a pregnant uterus. The most frequent complication reported in the study was weight gain which occurred in 23% of women at 6 or 12 months. Unfortunately, the study did not correlate the weight of the uterus removed with the amount of weight gained. In the fat volume equation, decreasing N will increase fat volume O. Their study is consistent with the hypothesis that intra-abdominal nonfat volume is a fat volume determining factor.

The radius of the stomach is the last parameter of the fat weight equation to discuss. Embryologically, the stomach begins at 5 weeks gestation as a fusiform dilatation of the intestinal tract. During gestation, the stomach reshapes and has a greater and lesser curvature. At any point on the surface of the stomach, two radii exist. By LaPlace's law, the larger radii will have the greater tension. The IGLE sensors in the neuromechanical model may sense both, and the greatest tension occurs at the largest radius.

Although no one has hypothesized that abnormalities of the stomach causes obesity, surgical therapy has been directed at modifying the stomach. Gastric banding was used to create a small volume stomach (approximately $50 \, cm^3$) at the fundus, with a small output for drainage. This operation was unsuccessful for several reasons. The pouch could expand over time and the contents did not create satiety because the IGLE sensors were not located within the pouch. Patients had difficulty digesting solid food and learned to eat liquids that passed rapidly through the small outlet.

Currently, one of the most effective weight loss operations is the gastric sleeve.[7] The sleeve reduces the volume capacity of the stomach to approximately $150 \, cm^3$, and the meal reaches the IGLE sensors within the antrum and corpus. The stomach is reshaped similar to a cylinder and any point on the wall has two radii. In one direction, the wall is curved but in the other direction the wall is almost a straight line. A straight line has an infinite radius. The gastric sleeve reduces the volume capacity of the stomach, changes the shape of the stomach, increases the radius r_s, and decreases the compliance of the stomach wall, and the IGLE sensors are exposed to increased tension. Fig. 6.4. Satiety is achieved with less meal volume, reducing weight. Appendix 6.1.

Gastric banding and gastric sleeve both decrease the volume capacity and compliance of the stomach. Gastric banding decreases the radius and gastric sleeve increases the radius. The IGLE are not exposed to the meal volume in gastric banding but are exposed in the gastric sleeve.

Comparison of Gastric Banding and Gastric Sleeve

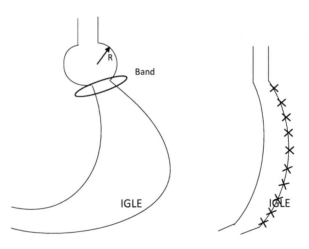

	Volume	Radius	IGLE Receptor
Gastric Band	$50 \, cm^3$	Decreased	Not Exposed
Gastric Sleeve	$150 \, cm^3$	Increased	Exposed

FIGURE 6.4

Comparison of gastric banding and gastric sleeve.

The gastric band has proven less effective, while the gastric sleeve is one of the most successful restrictive bariatric surgical operations. These human studies support the neuromechanical hypothesis and the fat volume equation $O = [(RC_a/Kr_s) - b_aC_a - N]/D$.

Appendix 6.1
Satiety equations after restrictive bariatric surgery for obesity

The satiety equations in Appendix 6.1 were used to determine the value of C_1 and C_2.

$$\text{where} \quad C1 = \frac{RA_B - KS_aNA_B - b_ar_sA_B - b_sr_sA_B}{1 + KS_aA_B + KS_sA_B}$$

$$C_2 = \frac{KS_aDA_{B'}}{1 + KS_aAB + KS_sA_B}$$

These are the correct values for all conditions.

Assuming obesity has occurred and a gastric restrictive operation has been performed, then the stiffness of the anterior abdominal wall is much less than the stiffness of the stomach wall ($S_s \gg S_a$); therefore, $KS_sA_B \gg KS_aA_B$ and KS_aA_B can be discarded. For the system to be F dominant, then $KS_sA_B \gg 1$, therefore 1 is also discarded, then

$$C_1 = \frac{R}{KS_s} - \frac{NS_a}{S_s} - \frac{b_ar_s}{KS_s} - \frac{b_sr_s}{KS_s}$$

$$C_2 = \frac{DS_a}{S_s}$$

Meal volume M after restrictive bariatric surgery

$$\frac{R - KNS_a - b_ar_s - b_sr_s - KDS_aO}{KS_s} = M_{restrictive}$$

$$\frac{RC_s}{r_sK} - \frac{NC_s}{C_a} - \frac{b_aC_s}{K} - \frac{b_aC_s}{K} - \frac{DC_s}{C_a}O = M_{restrictive}$$

This equation is difficult to interpret and the graphs in Figs. 6A.1, 6A.2, and 6A.3 display the changes in meal volume with decreased stomach compliance C_s and increase b_s after restrictive bariatric surgery.

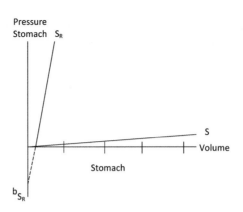

FIGURE 6A.1

Stomach volume pressure curve for a normal stomach S or for a stomach after gastric restrictive surgery S_R.

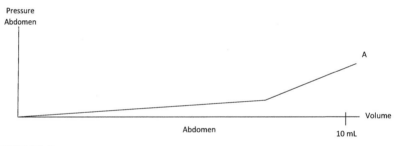

FIGURE 6A.2

Abdominal volume pressure curve for high compliance anterior abdominal wall.

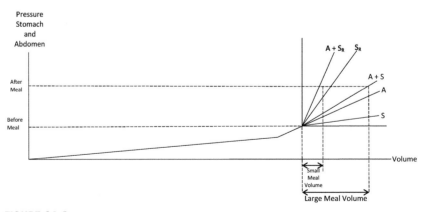

FIGURE 6A.3

Pressure volume curve from combining figures 6A.1 and 6A.2. The A + S curve includes the A and S components and requires a large meal volume. After gastric restrictive surgery, A + S_R curve include the A and S_R components and require a small meal volume.

References

1. Marques A, Brenda E, Pereira M, de Castro M, Abramo A. Plication of Abdominoplasties with Marlex mesh. *Ann Plast Surg*. 1995:117–134.
2. Koopman H. Internal signals cause changes in food Intake in one-way crossed intestinal rats. *Brain Res Bull*. 1985;14:595–603.
3. Dark J, Forger N, Zucker I. Rapid recovery of body mass after surgical removal of adipose tissue in ground squirrels. *Proc Natl Acad Sci USA*. April 1984;81:2270–2272.
4. Ersek R, Salisbury M, Girling R. Metabolic modulation by lipoplasty: a case report and invitation for investigators. *Aesthetic Plast Surg*. 2004;28:120–122.
5. *Developed by the National Center Fr Health Statistics in Collaboration with the National Center for Chronic Disease Prevention and Health Promotion*; 2000. Published May 30, 2000 http://www.cdc.gov/growthcharts.
6. Carlson K, Miller B, Fowler F. The Maine women's health study: I. Outcomes of hysterectomy. *Obstet Gynecol*. 1994;83(4):556–565.
7. Shoar S, Saber A. Long-term and midterm outcomes of laparoscopic sleeve gastrectomy versus Roux-en-Y gastric bypass: a systematic review and meta-analysis of comparative studies. *Surg Obes Relat Dis*. 2017;13:170–180.

Energy

Chapter outline

Abstract

Evolution requires survival, and survival requires energy storage. Although volume is sensed and weight is regulated, energy storage is essential for survival. Energy expenditure is divided into three components: resting (60%), nonresting (30%), and thermal (10%). Forcing dietary caloric changes in an attempt to change weight results in energy expenditure changes that oppose weight change. The pharmaceutical industry has had limited success in creating a medication that safely increases energy expenditure. Bariatric surgery does not increase energy expenditure. Obesity produces joint degeneration and cardiovascular disease that prevents physical exertion and increased energy expenditure. However, pulmonary energy consumption can increase 50-fold. Decreased abdominal capacity and decreased compliance of the abdominal wall (abdominoplasty with mesh reinforcement) increases pulmonary energy consumption and can be used to force the negative caloric balance required to reduce weight. Increasing expenditure to satisfy the requirements of breathing is essential.

Keywords: Negative caloric balance; Nonresting energy; Pulmonary energy expenditure; Resting energy; Second law of thermodynamics; Thermal energy.

Energy is required to maintain life. Without energy cells are unable to maintain their structural integrity and degenerate by the second law of thermodynamics. Stored fat can supply the energy required, when the external energy supply is interrupted. The average man has 20 pounds of fat that contain 72,000 kcals and can supply 2600 kcals per day for 28 days. More fat can be stored but has the disadvantage of additional weight. During evolution, a balance was achieved between the amount of fat stored to survive famine and the additional weight which limits man's ability to function efficiently and escape predators.

People are not cognizant of the caloric value of stored fat or it's volume but are aware of the weight, since it is easily measured by a scale. The human body cannot sense potential energy stored as fat, nor fat weight directly but can sense fat volume. Although we have focused on volume regulation to regulate weight, the purpose of the control system is to maintain energy reserves to ensure survival. Chemical energy is required for the biochemical reactions necessary for the neuromechanical dual closed loop to function and maintain stored fat energy. Consider an analogy to an electronic sound system shown in Fig. 7.1. The input is a record player that converts mechanical energy from motion of the stylus into electrical energy. The electrical signal is amplified and then sent to the speaker. The speaker converts the electrical energy back to mechanical energy, creating sound. The record player is the input, but the system will not function unless it is plugged into an electrical outlet to provide energy. The human energy regulating system is similar. We must be "plugged into" an energy source to provide energy to the control system. A wide variety of food serves as our energy source that allows man to regulate stored fat energy. The neuromechanical dual closed loop control system regulates energy when the caloric intake is greater than or equal to the caloric expenditure. Stored energy is not regulated when caloric expenditure is greater than the caloric intake.

Energy expenditure has been divided into three components. Resting energy is 60% of the total and supplies the requirements for cardiopulmonary

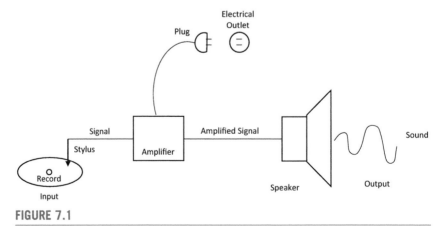

FIGURE 7.1

Record player sound system.

function and cellular maintenance. Thermal energy is 10% of the total and supplies the energy requirements for digestion, transportation, and deposit of nutrition. Nonresting energy is required for physical activity and it constitutes 30% of the total. Energy studies were performed on normal weight and obese patients who were overfed or underfed to force weight increases or decreases, respectively.[1] The results of the study show that energy expenditure changes to oppose the forced weight changes. When obese patients are forced to lose weight by dietary reduction, total energy expenditure decreases and attempts to return the weight to its original value.

Energy is required to perform work. Pulmonary work performed by the diaphragm, during inspiration, is mathematically defined as work $W = \int P\, dV$, which corresponds to the area under the pressure volume curves. In Fig. 7.2, the work of diaphragmatic breathing 0.5 L, in normal weight, forced overweight and forced underweight is the hatched area under the curve. Energy consumption is greatest for the forced overweight and least for the forced underweight in both normal and obese subjects. These findings are consistent with Dr. Leibel's study of forced overweight increases energy consumption to return weight to the original value and forced underweight decreases energy consumption to return weight to original value.

Now consider normal, normal forced overweight and acquired obesity from increased compliance and capacity in Fig. 7.3. Acquired obesity requires less energy for diaphragmatic breathing 0.5 L than normal weight, which requires less than normal forced overweight. Strenuous exercise

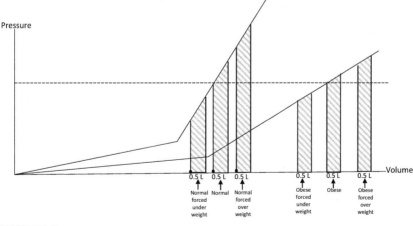

FIGURE 7.2

Pressure volume curve for normal, obese and after forced overweight or underweight.
The striped area represents the work of breathing 0.5 Liters.

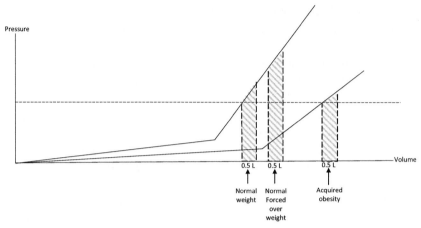

FIGURE 7.3

Pressure volume curve for normal weight, normal weight forced overweight, and acquired obesity.
The striped area represents the work of breathing 0.5 Liters.

requires diaphragmatic breathing, and clinical studies show obese patients use less energy to perform strenuous work than normal weight patients.

Is it possible to increase energy expenditure despite decreasing weight? The pharmaceutical industry has been searching for a pill that increases energy expenditure with limited success. Bariatric surgery does not increase energy expenditure. Unfortunately, people with long durational obesity frequently have joint degeneration or cardiovascular disease that prevents physical exertion, therefore, they are unable to increase nonresting energy expenditure. When less food is consumed, thermal energy will decrease. The last option is increasing resting energy. Resting energy is the largest portion of the total energy and supplies the requirements for cardiopulmonary function. Is it possible to safely increase cardiopulmonary energy demands? Normal respiration consumes only 3%–5% of total energy expenditure (80–130 Kcals in a 70 kg man), but this can increase 50-fold with exertion (3900–6500 Kcals). The energy required for respiration will be increased if the chest wall has decreased compliance or the diaphragm works against increased abdominal pressure.

Now consider energy consumption in acquired obesity, normal weight, and acquired obesity after abdominoplasty with mesh reinforcement. Fig. 7.4. Acquired obesity has decreased work of breathing compared to normal. Abdominoplasty with mesh reinforcement reduces abdominal capacity and wall compliance, increases intra-abdominal pressure, and increases the work required for diaphragmatic breathing. Abdominoplasty with mesh reinforcement also decreases the compliance of the rib cage

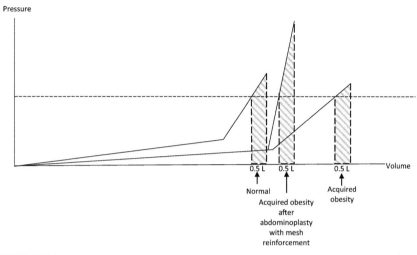

FIGURE 7.4

Pressure volume curve for normal, acquired obesity and acquired obesity after abdominoplasty with mesh reinforcement.
The striped area represents the work of breathing 0.5 Liters.

which increases the work for chest breathing. Obese people will increase energy expenditure to satisfy the work requirements for breathing. Decreased compliance of the abdominal wall and capacity of the abdomen can be used to produce the negative caloric balance that is required for weight loss in obese patients with normal pulmonary function.

Reference

1. Leibel R, Rosenbaum M, Hirsch J. Changes in energy expenditure resulting from altered body weight. *N Engl J Med.* 1995;332:621−627.

Evolution and memes

Chapter outline

Abstract

Eating has been programmed by our DNA for survival. The question is, how do we know when to stop? Meal volume is fed back to the hypothalamus and compared with the reference volume to determine hunger or satiety. Up to this point, evolution has determined the control system. Man has uniquely evolved, and our minds set us apart from all other specifies. Memes are cultural information units that are transferred into the mind, from person to person, but are not genetic. Simultaneous with the acquired obesity epidemic, our memes have changed. Manual labor is undesirable, physical fitness is nonessential, instant gratification from high fat foods is pleasurable, and obesity has become acceptable. In our weight control system, hunger or satiety signals are transferred to the cortical processor that is under mind control. Normally, hunger induces eating and satiety terminates the meal. Memes determine the outcome and can alter the cortical processor's response.

Keywords: Amoeba; Anorexia nervosa; Control process; Cultural information; Darwin's tree of life; Evolution; Manual labor; Meme; Physical fitness; Tensile strength; Truth table.

Eating, surviving, and reproducing are essential components for continued evolution. The second law of thermodynamics requires closed systems, such as living organisms, to acquire exogenous energy for survival. In humans, food is our energy source. Newborns eat immediately, because eating is not learned but programmed by our DNA. The question is not why we eat, but how do we know when to stop? Consider a unicellular organism, the ameba. They eat by forming pseudopods from the surface that surround food in a vacuole, which is digested. How does an ameba know when to stop eating? The ameba's DNA determines the tensile strength of the external cell wall. When amebas acquire food and increase volume, they assume a spherical shape which has the maximum volume for the least surface area. At this point, the tension of the cell wall mechanically prevents pseudopods from forming. Satiety is achieved by increased tension on the external cell wall. Fig. 8.1.

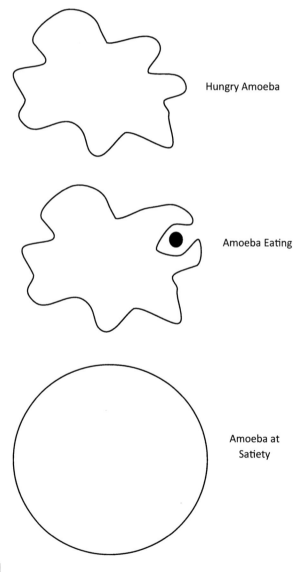

Hungry Amoeba

Amoeba Eating

Amoeba at Satiety

FIGURE 8.1

Amoeba shapes.

Since man has evolved from simpler life forms, are there similarities to the ameba? The human stomach wall can be considered analogous to an ameba. Food is topologically outside the body when it enters the inside of the stomach. With the volume increase of a meal, the intragastric pressure and intra-abdominal pressure increases the stomach wall tension. The IGLE tension receptors respond by generating electrical signals and use pulse frequency modulation to transmit through the vagus nerve to the nucleus tractus solitarius. The nucleus tractus solitarius then transfers the signal to the hypothalamus and satiety is achieved when the feedback volume sensed exceeds the internal reference volume. Fig. 5.4 The hypothalamus signals the cortex that satiety is achieved. The cortex controls the upper extremity motion required for feeding. Man's upper extremities are analogues to the ameba pseudopods. DNA determines satiety but the cortex has ultimate control of eating.

Man has uniquely evolved, and we have a mind that sets us apart from all other species. Other species eat to satiety and then stop. Animals that eat beyond satiety become overweight or obese, are at an evolutionary disadvantage, and are devoured by predators. Domesticated animals can be overfed because their owners protect them. Man's mind is unique and capable of conscious foresight. During our evolution, it was of survival advantage to overeat in preparation for predictable periods of decreased food supply. However, this also allows the mind to ignore satiety. In America, the classic example is the Thanksgiving Day feast. People ignore satiety and eat for pleasure to the point of abdominal pain or pulmonary compromise. This is a common behavior that has spread throughout American and can be considered a meme. Meme is short for mimeme, which was first described in 1976 by Richard Dakin in his book, *The Selfish Gene*.[1] Memes are cultural information units that are transmitted from person to person but are not genetic. In Darwin's tree of life, DNA slowly propagates vertically but memes rapidly propagate horizontally. Fig. 8.2 Memes spread from mind to mind, altering behavior faster and with a wider ranging than genetic changes.

Obese children were rare in previous generations. As a child, I remember one individual who was fat in high school and was ridiculed as fat Pat. In 2017, the authors spent a month visiting China. Upon our return to America, after seeing only thin Chinese, we were shocked by the rampant obesity in America, that previously went unnoticed. Fortunately, or unfortunately, our current generations have become tolerant of obesity and our meme has changed. Another meme that has changed is the

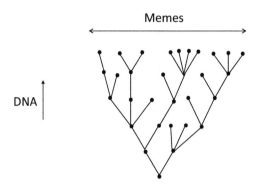

FIGURE 8.2

Darwin's tree of life.

concept of working smarter not harder. During college, I worked one summer doing manual labor at the same factory my father and grandfather worked. This reinforced the importance of education and avoiding manual labor. The current generations do less manual labor than the past generations and physical fitness has consequently declined. Physical education has also been eliminated from many school curriculums. These changes have spread rapidly throughout the world and established a new meme.

Memes may also change that to reduce the incidence of obesity. Improved women's rights allow the current generations of women to choose to have less children or have no children at all. Adoption is an acceptable alternative used by many women today. In Chapter 9, the association of obesity with pregnancy, especially multiple pregnancies, will be described. Current women's fashion emphasizes thin, gaunt, sticklike models as their ideal. This has generated memes in women that may become pathological with anorexia nervosa as an extreme example. These memes prohibit eating despite hunger.

Memes act within the neuromechanical control system. In Fig. 8.3, the cortical processor is located between the hypothalamus and the motor cortex. Fig. 5.4 displays hunger and satiety generation. When the feedback volume is greater than reference volume, satiety occurs. When feedback volume is less than reference volume, hunger persists. The hunger or satiety signals are sent through the cortical processor that is controlled by the meme. The input output truth table for the cortical processor is

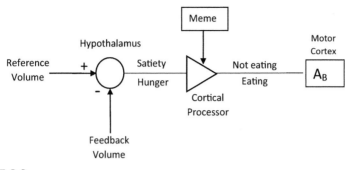

FIGURE 8.3

Satiety and hunger signals generated by the hypothalamus are processed in the cortex controlled by memes.

Truth Table for the Cortical Processor

	Input	Output
Over Eating Meme (Example Thanksgiving)	Satiety Hunger	Eating Eating
Normal Meme	Satiety Hunger	Not Eating Eating
Under Eating Meme (Example Anorexia Nervosa)	Satiety Hunger	Not Eating Not Eating

FIGURE 8.4

Truth table for the cortical processor.

shown in Fig. 8.4. Normally, the signal from the hypothalamus passes through the cortical processor with satiety terminating a meal, but hunger requires eating. If the meme ignores satiety, then the output is eating. If the meme ignores hunger, food is not consumed, and the output is satiety. The incidence of acquired obesity has increased simultaneously with our changing memes. DNA changes are slow and cannot occur in a few generations. Satiety is determined by DNA, but memes can alter the mind's response.

Reference

1. Dawkins R. *The Selfish Gene*. NY: Oxford University Press; 1989.

Acquired obesity

Chapter outline

Abstract

The neuromechanical model can be used to explain the etiology of acquired obesity. The feedback signal that creates satiety originates in the IGLE receptors within the stomach wall, from tension generated by pressure within the stomach wall and the abdominal cavity. Intra-abdominal pressure is generated by intra-abdominal volume within the anterior abdominal wall. Abdominal wall compliance depends on the mechanical strength of its muscle and fascia. Muscle strength depends on its length and physical fitness. Fascia is elastic and is analogous to a spring. When a spring is overstretched and exceeds its elastic modulus, irreversible damage occurs. The mechanical failure cycle begins with decreased mechanical strength of the abdominal wall that requires increased intra-abdominal fat to achieve satiety. The increased fat stretches the muscle and fascia, resulting in additional loss of mechanical strength. This cycle repeats, resulting in acquired obesity. Irreversible acquired obesity occurs when fascia is stretched beyond its elastic modulus, resulting in irreversible damage.

Keywords: Abdominal capacity; Abdominal wall compliance; Acquired obesity; Elastic modulus; IGLE receptors; Irreversible obesity; LaPlace's law; Mechanical failure cycle; Mechanical strength of muscle and fascia; Obesity; Physical fitness; Reversible obesity; Starling's law.

Human and animal research has proven genetic causes of obesity. These are rare, described in detail in standard textbooks, and are not the subject of this book. Instead, we will focus on the worldwide epidemic of acquired obesity. In the previous chapters, control system theory, human studies, and animal experiments were used to derive the neuromechanical hypothesis

Weight Regulation and Curing Acquired Obesity. https://doi.org/10.1016/B978-0-323-77854-1.00009-3

for weight regulation. The neuromechanical model, Fig. 5.3, has three divisions: neuro, neuromechanical, and mechanical. The neuro division is located within the brain and is connected by nerves to the periphery. An acquired disease that affects the brain would likely produce neurological symptoms, but these have not been observed with acquired obesity. Diabetes is an acquired disease that decreases nerve conduction. The vagus nerve is damaged resulting in decreased feedback. Type II diabetics have a 60%−90% incident of obesity which requires treatment to return conduction to normal, increase feedback, and cure obesity. Diabetes is an acquired disease that can cause obesity but is not the cause of the current epidemic, since the vast majority of acquired obesity patients are not diabetic.

The second division to consider is neuromechanical. The pylorus is a neuromechanical switch that is controlled by the vagus nerve and can be adversely affected by diabetes, resulting in delayed gastric emptying. This may prolong the slow cycle but would not create obesity. An acquired disease specific to the IGLE tension receptors could exist but has never been reported. However, with aging, the IGLE tension receptors are known to degenerate in rats.[1] This may increase weight with aging but does not explain acquired obesity. The third and last division to consider is mechanical. A biological neuromechanical control system is analogous to a man-made electromechanical control system. The etiology of a failed electromechanical control system is frequently mechanical. In general, mechanical components wear out sooner than electrical components. The question is, which component within the mechanical division fails and how does it cause obesity?

The neuromechanical hypothesis was discussed in Chapter 5 and was illustrated in Fig. 5.3. When feedback is decreased, weight increases, regulation decreases, and weight becomes increasingly dietary dependent. With complete loss of negative feedback, the closed loop control system degenerates into an open loop control system and is totally dietary dependent. The feedback signal originates within the wall of the stomach from the IGLE tension receptors.[2] Tension within the wall of the stomach is determined by the meal volume, stomach wall compliance, and radius of the stomach. Tension on the outside wall of the stomach is determined by intra-abdominal volume, abdominal wall compliance, and the radius of the stomach. The compliance of the anterior abdominal wall is a significant factor determining feedback.

The compliance of the anterior abdominal wall is dependent on the mechanical strength of the fascia and muscle. Since the muscle and fascia of the anterior abdominal wall are not homogeneous, the tension on the internal surface varies. Because of the nonhomogenous mechanical strength and mechanical load, wall failure occurs at specific locations. Hernias represent complete mechanical failure of both muscle and fascia of the wall and are one of the most common pathological conditions requiring surgery. The abdominal wall must create pressure to balance intra-abdominal pressure. LaPlace's Law states that pressure = tension/radius. An abdominal wall with decreased mechanical strength generates less tension; therefore, the radius must decrease to compensate. When weakened, the normally flat abdominal wall bulges anteriorly, decreasing the radius. This is always observed in obesity. Muscle strength depends on physical fitness and muscle length. When the muscle has decreased mechanical strength, the fascia is exposed to increased mechanical loading and stretches. Fascial strength depends on connective tissue biology but can be irreversibly weakened by extension beyond its elastic modulus. Figs. 9.1 and 9.2 showed a set of five springs; unstretched, three with progressive increased stretching, and one overstretched. When a spring is stretched beyond its elastic modulus, the spring undergoes internal fracture, mechanical failure, and never returns to its original length. The spring is irreversibly damaged.

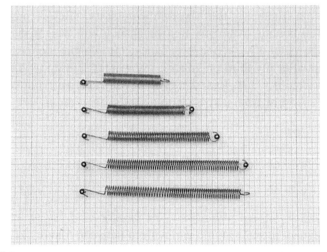

FIGURE 9.1

Stretched springs.

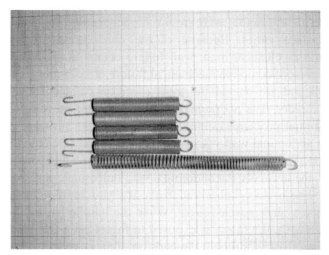

FIGURE 9.2

Reversible and Irreversible stretched springs.

Acquired obesity is caused by physiologic or meme changes in men, women, and children. The etiology of physiologic acquired obesity is easiest to understand in postpartum women. Medical research has discovered that 73% of obese women attribute their obesity to pregnancy.[3] Studies in primates reveal 10% weight gain after pregnancy.[4] As a plastic surgeon, I am frequently told the following story. "Before pregnancy, I weighed 120 pounds. After my first pregnancy, my weight increased to 135 pounds. After my second pregnancy, my weight increased to 160 pounds. But after my third pregnancy, my weight shot up to 200 pounds. I have modified my diet, joined a gym, began exercising but still weigh 195 pounds. I went from a size six to a size sixteen dress."

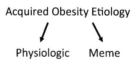

The pregnant uterus volume varies from between 5 and 20 L. Volume expansion within the abdominal containment system stretches the anterior abdominal wall. The age of the woman, pregnant uterus volume, and physical properties of her muscle and fascia determine compliance.

Postpartum, the stretched abdominal wall has increased compliance and more intra-abdominal volume is required to achieve satiety. For example, assume the abdominal cavity now requires one additional liter of volume, compared to before pregnancy, to achieve satiety. Using the distribution ratio D of 0.2 for women, then 1 L of additional intra-abdominal fat would require 5 L of total fat or 10 pounds of fat. Each pregnancy begins at a higher intra-abdominal volume and the pregnant uterus causes additional muscle and fascial stretching. A series of pregnancies, with intra-abdominal volume expansion and progressive increased abdominal wall compliance, may produce obesity.[5]

Nonpregnant women, adult men, and children become obese by a similar physiologic mechanism. Society has moved from the industrial age to the information age and physical activity has been reduced. The information age has also become the entertainment age and children entertain themselves passively, instead of actively with physical exertion. The progressive loss of muscle strength in adults, or failure to increase muscle strength in growing children, increases abdominal wall compliance, decreases the feedback, and requires additional intra-abdominal fat to achieve satiety. The increased mechanical load stretches the abdominal wall, lengthens the muscle decreasing muscular strength by Starling's law. The fascia stretches to compensate for loss of muscle strength, is progressively weakened, and may exceed its elastic modulus. Unless the cycle is interrupted, progressive mechanical changes produce obesity Fig. 9.3.

The second etiology of acquired obesity is memes. In 1994,[6] Pasquet and Apfelbaum published a human study in young Cameroonian men who participated in a 4- to 6-month cultural tradition of overfeeding called guru, a meme. Fat weight before, at completion of guru, and 30 months after completion of guru were 7.9 ± 2.4 kg, 19.7 ± 3.6 kg, and 9.0 ± 2.9 kg, respectively. Obesity was reversed after returning to the original meme and not eating beyond satiety. The neuromechanical model in Fig. 5.3 is genetically determined but required termination of eating when satiety is achieved. These young Cameroonian men have changed their response to satiety and overeat because of the guru meme. Eating is pleasurable and many people chose to eat beyond satiety. This is not a physical cause of obesity, but over time obesity can change the physiology creating obesity indistinguishable from physiologic obesity.

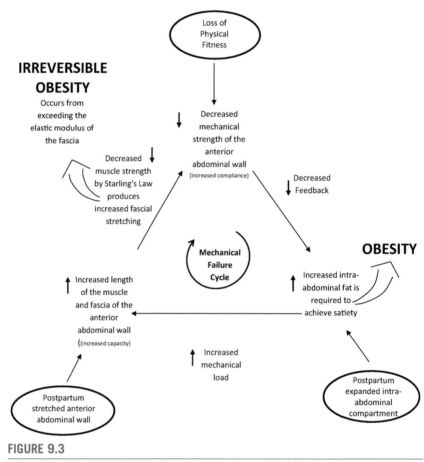

FIGURE 9.3

Mechanical failure cycle.

   Human studies and animal experiments prove that there are two pathological types of acquired obesity, reversible and irreversible.[7] Obesity was induced in rats by feeding them a high fat diet. After 17 weeks, a subset of obese rats were returned to a standard laboratory diet (low fat) and obesity was reversed. After 30 weeks, a second subset of rats were returned to a standard laboratory diet; however, the obesity did not reverse. Multiple human studies have shown that diet alone frequently fails to reverse obesity. Both animal experiments and human studies show the existence of reversible and irreversible obesity.

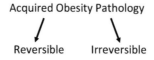

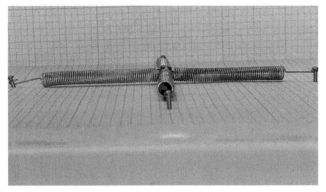

FIGURE 9.4

2-Dimensional stretched springs.

Acquired obesity may progress to mechanical deterioration of the muscle and fascia of the anterior abdominal wall. The abdominal wall is a two-dimensional structure, and Figs. 9.4 and 9.5 show two-dimensional springs, stretched and overstretched. When the springs are stretched beyond the elastic modulus, they undergo mechanical failure and never return to normal. The springs also create a hemispherical space that increases volume capacity. Similarly, irreversible obesity results from stretching the abdominal fascia beyond its elastic modulus which increases compliance and capacity.

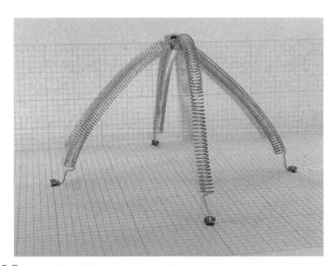

FIGURE 9.5

2-Dimensional irreversible stretched springs (Note: increased volume capacity).

What happens to the dual closed loop control system in the extreme case of total mechanical failure of the anterior abdominal wall? With total mechanical failure, the values of b_a and S_a decrese to zero. The neuromechanical model previously shown in Fig. 5.1 changes and is now shown in Fig. 9.6 with S_a and b_a removed. As a result, the dual closed loop becomes a single closed loop and an open loop as shown in Fig. 9.7.

The closed loop determines the meal volume. Since Since R, A_B, b_s, r_s, and S_s are fixed values, that do not vary with the food eaten, then meal volume is constant. However, fat volume is $A_C A_A$ times the meal volume. Since A_C varies depending on the food eaten, then fat volume is not regulated. Fast cycle satiety is achieved within the closed loop when food is within the stomach. After the food has left the stomach and entered the intestines, slow satiety is not achieved since the slow closed loop has been interrupted. Patients will experience satiety when eating and shortly thereafter while the stomach empties. Without slow satiety, hunger is only eliminated by eating and patients will eat almost continuously. This phenomenon was observed in the bedridden, 450-pound patient discussed in the end of Chapter 2.

Complete loss of negative feedback is rare. The more common form of acquired obesity is a combination of low F and high A which results in AF much greater than one. Weight is regulated at 1/F, but since F is low obesity occurs. This combination was described in the 240-pound patient from Chapter 2 (page 12) and is difficult to treat by diet, since obese patients prefer high fat foods.

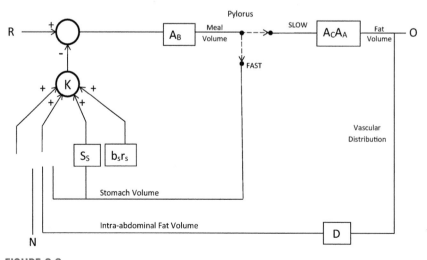

FIGURE 9.6

Complete mechanical failure of the anterior abdominal wall eliminates S_a and b_a is zero.

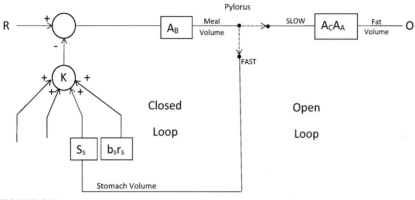

FIGURE 9.7

Complete Mechanical Failure of the Anterior Abdominal Wall.

1. The dual closed loops become one closed loop and one open loop.
2. Meal volume is regulated.
3. Fat volume is not regulated and depends on meal volume, A_C and A_A.
4. Fast cycle satiety remains but slow cycle satiety is eliminated.
5. Hunger returns rapidly at the end of the fast cycle resulting in continuous eating.

References

1. Phillips R, Walter G, Powley T. Age-related changes in vagal afferents innervating the gastrointestinal tract. *Auton Neurosci: Basic Clin.* 2010;153:90−98.
2. Piessevaux H, Tack J, Wilmer A, Coulie B, Geubel A, Janssens J. Perception of changes in wall tension of the proximal stomach in humans. *Gut.* 2001;49: 203−208.
3. Linne Y, Barkeling B, Rossner S. Long-term weight development after pregnancy. *Obes Rev.* 2002;3:75−83.
4. Riopelle AJ, Shell WF. Protein deprovation in primates. XI Determinates of weight change during and after pregnancy. *Am J Clin Nutr.* 1978;31: 394−400.
5. Williamson D, Madans J, Pamuk E, Flegal K, Kendrick J, Serdula M. A prospective study of childbearing and 10-year weight gain in US white women 25 to 45 years of age. *Int J Obes.* 1994;18:561−569.
6. Pasquet P, Apfelbaum M. Recovery of initial body weight and composition after long-term massive overfeeding in men1-3. *Am J Clin Nutr.* 1994;60: 861−863.
7. Hill J, Dorton J, Sykes M, Digirolamo M. Reversal of dietary obesity is influenced by its duration and severity. *Int J Obes.* 1989;13:711−722.

Curing acquired obesity

Chapter outline

Abstract

Knowledge of the physiology of weight regulation and the pathology of the acquired obesity is essential for prevention, treatment, and cure. The transition from normal weight to overweight to obesity can be prevented by diet, physical fitness, and changed memes. The most effective current treatments for acquired obesity are bariatric surgery using gastric restriction, intestinal malabsorption, or both. These treatments do not cure acquired obesity, since the cause is not an enlarged stomach or excessive intestinal length. Curing irreversible acquired obesity requires increased mechanical strength of the anterior abdominal wall. Strength is increased by abdominoplasty with mesh reinforcement, directly from the mesh and indirectly by Starling's law's effect on muscle. In cases of extreme obesity, a bariatric surgical procedure may be used as an adjuvant initially, allowing safe performance of an abdominoplasty with mesh reinforcement later.

Keywords: Abdominoplasty with mesh reinforcement; Bariatric surgery; Caloric value determination; Compliance of the stomach; Control system parameters; Core exercises; Dietary education; Liposuction; Low fat diet; Malabsorption or combined; Modified feedback; Negative caloric balance; Pathology of acquired obesity; Physical education; Prevention; Radius of stomach; Restrictive; Reversible versus irreversible obesity; Treatment versus cure; Work of breathing.

A disease cannot be cured without knowledge of the normal physiology and the pathological changes. The new concepts of the neuromechanical hypothesis replace the misconceptions of sensing total body fat biochemically

Weight Regulation and Curing Acquired Obesity. https://doi.org/10.1016/B978-0-323-77854-1.00010-X

and that the stomach senses only intragastric volume. The neuromechanical hypothesis is supported by anatomic and physiologic studies of IGLE tension receptors, the stomach brain neurologic connections, and abdominal compliance and capacity. A unified theory of weight control has been elucidated, which is capable of predicting weight with variations of the control system parameters. Physiologic acquired obesity resulted from changes in the control system parameters, not control system failure. Meme acquired obesity occurs from ignoring satiety generated by a normal control system.

Patients and physicians must be educated to prevent acquired obesity. Prevention requires recognition of the pathological transition from the normal weight to overweight and finally to obesity. Early intervention is best to prevent the cycle of decreased abdominal wall strength, increased intra-abdominal fat, and stretched muscle and fascia, which eventually creates irreversible obesity. In children, the parents, physicians, and schools are obligated to prevent acquired obesity. Children must be educated to the wide variations of fat content in foods. They need to be directed away from high fat foods and toward low fat foods, such as fruits and vegetables. Children naturally eat to satiety and terminate eating, a normal meme. They should not be forced to eat beyond satiety and create an abnormal meme to satisfy their parent's, the food industry's, or the restaurant industry's misconceptions of meal size. Physical education, particularly core exercises designed to increase abdominal wall muscle strength, is essential to prevent acquired obesity. In adults, low levels of education have been associated with increased prevalence of obesity.[1] Likewise, they must be educated to the wide variations of fat content in food, to make proper selections and the importance of core exercise to maintain abdominal wall muscle tone and prevent acquired obesity. In adult males, alcoholism has been shown to be associated with acquired obesity.[1] This may be due to central nervous system depression, with decreased sensation of satiety leading to volume overloading. Education on alcohol abuse is essential. Restaurants also encourage eating beyond satiety by providing larger-sized meals. Bringing the dessert tray to customers after they have consumed a meal is a technique used to optimize profits, but encourages overeating. "There is always room for dessert" meme should be eliminated. Adults eat beyond satiety to the point of reflux and routinely use antacids, rather than decreasing meal volume. Adults must reestablish the normal meme of terminating meals at satiety. Pulmonary compromise is the ultimate terminator of overeating, when satiety is ignored. Nothing exceeds the joy of breathing. Multiparas women are at high risk for obesity due to progressive volume expansion and anterior abdominal wall damage.[2]

It is the obstetrician's obligation to monitor weight and provide dietary advice during the pregnancy. After the pregnancy, women need to make the necessary dietary changes, establish their original meme, and resume core physical exercises to reduce postpartum weight.

Treatment of acquired obesity is more difficult than prevention. Current obesity therapy is divided into dietary, medical, and surgical. Dietary studies have shown that low caloric and low fat diets can reduce weight, but none have proven superior, despite celebrity endorsement claims. Satiety is achieved by volume loading. The caloric density of food (calories/volume) is $8.1 \, kcal/cm^3$ of fat, $5.4 \, kcal/cm^3$ of protein, and $6.2 \, kcal/cm^3$ of carbohydrates Appendix 10.1. The lowest caloric diet has the lowest fat content. Medical treatment has been directed toward decreasing fat absorption, increasing energy expenditure, or achieving early satiety. This is despite the fact that there is no proof that acquired obesity occurs from increased fat absorption or from decreased metabolism. Multiple medications are available that can decrease weight, but none reverse the pathology of acquired obesity.

Currently, the most effective treatment for obesity has been surgical. Bariatric surgery is reserved for patients with BMI $>35 \, kg/m^2$ with medical conditions or BMI $>40 \, kg/m^2$ without. Bariatric surgery has been divided into restrictive, malabsorption, or combination. Restrictive surgery reduces the volume capacity of the stomach, which reduces meal volume Appendix 6.1. The malabsorption operations bypass segments of the small intestine, decreasing absorption of fat which decreases A_A. Five-year follow-up studies have shown that bariatric surgery techniques reduce excessive weight by approximately 70% in the first 2 years, but rebound gain occurs and the reduction at 5 years is approximately 55% of the excess weight.[3] These techniques are the standard of care today, despite the fact that no one has hypothesized that obesity is caused by an enlarged stomach or excessive small intestinal length. These operations create abnormal physiology in the stomach or small intestines that results in weight loss.

Fig. 10.1 displays the changes that bariatric surgery creates in the neuromechanical model. Malabsorption surgery decreases the absorption of fat A_A, which reduces the amplification of the slow loop. For a closed loop control system to regulate the output, the mathematical product of A times F must be much greater than 1. Any operation that decreases the amplification will decrease the product AF. Since irreversible acquired obesity is the result of decreased F, reducing A further reduces the product AF and the control system becomes increasingly dependent on the A value. The control system transforms from F dominant to codominant and finally to A

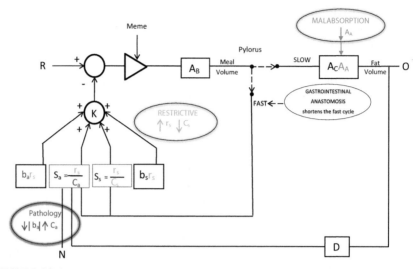

FIGURE 10.1

Pathological parameters in acquired obesity (Red), parameters changed with restrictive bariatric surgery (Green), malabsorptive bariatric surgery (Blue).

dominant with decreasing A values. Malabsorption bariatric surgery results in weight loss but not weight regulation. Weight becomes dependent on the fat content of the diet, but unfortunately obese patients like high fat diets. Malabsorption surgery does not reverse the pathological changes of acquired obesity and does not cure acquired obesity.

The gastric sleeve increases the radius of the stomach r_s and decreases the compliance of the stomach C_s. The result is increased feedback in the fast loop which creates satiety with less meal volume. Fat volume is determined by the slow loop and the increased value of r_s, increases the value of S_a, which increases feedback and the product AF. The goal is to increase AF so that it is much greater than 1 for the system to regulate weight. Increased F results in weight loss and improves weight regulation. The pathology of irreversible acquired obesity is mechanical failure of the anterior abdominal wall which increases C_a. Restrictive bariatric surgery does not reverse the pathological changes of irreversible acquired obesity and does not cure obesity. However, restrictive bariatric surgery increases the value of F and AF, which is superior to malabsorption bariatric surgery which decreases the value of A and AF.

There is a significant difference between treating a disease and curing the disease. Insulin is used in the treatment of diabetes but does not cure diabetes. Bariatric surgery is a treatment for obesity, but not the cure. Curing a disease requires therapy directed at the underlying cause. Physicians can educate obese patients about the importance of lowering the fat in the diet, exercising, terminating meals at satiety, and changing the meme, but it's ultimately dependent on patient cooperation. However, physicians can surgically modify feedback. Curing obesity requires the combined efforts of an educated, cooperative patient willing to restore a normal meme, and possibly operation(s) to reverse the underlying pathology.

It is possible to reverse acquired obesity by a combination of dietary fat reduction, changed meme, and increased feedback. Feedback has several components including abdominal wall compliance and fat distribution. Physical exercise that increases abdominal wall muscle strength increases feedback. Dietary fat reduction can result in weight reduction in obesity. If diet, exercise, and changing memes do not cure obesity, then the least invasive surgical procedure to increase feedback would be liposuction.[4] Liposuction decreases the extra-abdominal fat, increases the fat distribution ratio D, which increases feedback. The difference between the patient's weight and the desired weight will determine the volume of fat needed for removal. Liposuction is limited to approximately 5 liters or 10 pounds for outpatient surgery. Larger volumes can be done as inpatient surgery but with a higher complication rate. Liposuction can also be repeated to produce sequential weight loss. Depending on the patient's goals and current BMI, liposuction may not be appropriate. If the combination of dietary change, meme change, exercise, and liposuction would not be effective, then the next step would be surgical intervention to change the compliance and capacity of the abdomen. This is required for irreversible obesity due to abdominal wall damage. Abdominoplasty with mesh reinforcement has been discussed previously and, in my experience, has the capability to reduce BMI by 3.5 kg/m^2 in patients with a BMI greater than 30 kg/m^2. This procedure can also be done simultaneously with liposuction in order to eliminate two separate operations. In patients with a BMI greater than 35 kg/m^2, I recommend bariatric surgery instead of abdominoplasty with mesh reinforcement. Successful bariatric surgery reduces approximately 70% of the extra fat weight.[3] When the patient reaches their weight nadir, abdominoplasty with mesh reinforcement will achieve multiple goals. Excess hanging skin and fat are resected resulting in esthetic improvement and additional weight removal. The mesh decreases abdominal wall compliance and the capacity of the abdomen which may prevent rebound weight gain. Increased intra-abdominal pressure and decreased compliance of the anterior abdominal wall increase the work of breathing, resulting in the caloric deficit to reduce weight. Performing an abdominoplasty with mesh reinforcement after weight loss is technically easier and associated with less complications since the fat layer of the abdominal wall is thinner. If necessary, liposuction can be performed prior to the abdominoplasty with mesh reinforcement if the fat layer of the abdominal wall is still too thick. The goal of these procedures is to safely and permanently reverse the pathological changes in the parameters that determine weight.

Everyone should be educated to the basic principles of weight regulation, satiety meme, the wide range of fat content of food, and the importance of core exercises to maintain abdominal wall strength. Acquired obesity patients must consume a reduced fat diet, maintain an exercise program when possible, and if necessary, change their meme prior to surgical intervention. An acquired obesity treatment algorithm is provided in Fig. 10.2.

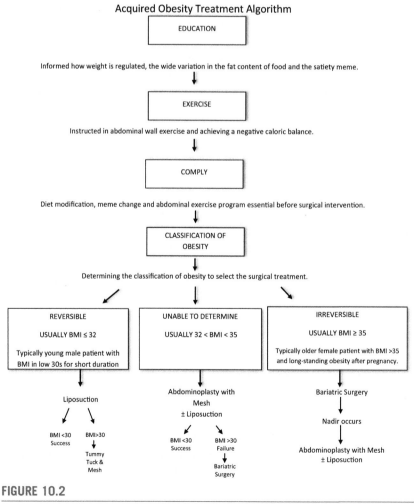

FIGURE 10.2

Acquired obesity treatment algorithm.

Appendix 10.1
Caloric volume density

Density is defined as weight divided by volume $\text{Density} = \dfrac{\text{grams}}{\text{cm}^3}$

$$\text{Fat} = \dfrac{0.9\text{g}}{\text{cm}^3}$$

$$\text{Protein} = \dfrac{1.35\text{g}}{\text{cm}^3}$$

$$\text{Carbohydrate} = \dfrac{1.54\text{g}}{\text{cm}^3}$$

Caloric weight density is energy divided by grams Caloric Weight Density $= \dfrac{\text{Kcal}}{\text{cm}^3}$

$$\text{Fat} = \dfrac{9\text{kcal}}{\text{g}}$$

$$\text{Protein} = \dfrac{4\text{Kcal}}{\text{g}}$$

$$\text{Carbohydrate} = \dfrac{4\text{Kcal}}{\text{g}}$$

Caloric volume density is energy divided by volume Caloric Volume Density $= \dfrac{\text{Kcal}}{\text{cm}^3}$

Caloric volume density is calculated by multiplying density times caloric weight density

$$\text{Fat}\ \dfrac{0.9\text{g}}{\text{cm}^3}\ \times\ \dfrac{9\text{Kcal}}{\text{g}}\ =\ \dfrac{8.1\text{Kcal}}{\text{cm}^3}$$

$$\text{Protein}\ \dfrac{1.35\text{g}}{\text{cm}^3}\ \times\ \dfrac{4\text{Kcal}}{\text{g}}\ =\ \dfrac{5.4\text{Kal}}{\text{cm}^3}$$

$$\text{Carbohydrate}\ \dfrac{1.54\text{g}}{\text{cm}^3}\ \times\ \dfrac{4\text{Kcal}}{\text{g}}\ =\ \dfrac{6.2\text{Kcal}}{\text{cm}^3}$$

Fat has the highest K calories per volume and protein has the lowest.

References

1. Rissanen AM, Heliovaara M, Knekt P, Reunanen A, Aromaa A. Determinants of weight gain and overweigh in adult Finns. *Eur J Clin Nutr.* 1991;45: 419–430.
2. Williamson D, Madans J, Pamuk E, Flegal k, Kendrick J, Serdula M. A prospective study of childbearing and 10-year weight gain in US white women 25 to 45 years of age. *Int J Obes.* 1994;18:561–569.
3. Benotti P, Forse R. The role of gastric surgery in the multidisciplinary management of severe obesity. *Am J Surg.* 1995;169:361–367.
4. Ersek R, Salisbury M, Girling R. Metabolic modulation by lipoplasty: a case report and invitation for investigators. *Aesthetic Plast Surg.* 2004;28: 120–122.

The future

11

Chapter outline

Abstract

Additional animal experiments and human studies can be performed to verify the neuromechanical hypothesis. Abdominal wall compliance measurements will be used to distinguish irreversible acquired obesity from reversible acquired obesity. Reversible acquired obesity can be treated with diet, exercise, changed memes, and less invasive surgery, possibly liposuction, intra-abdominal fat transfer, or abdominoplasty with mesh reinforcement. Irreversible acquired obesity always requires abdominoplasty with mesh reinforcement, but may necessitate adjuvant surgery first. Adjuvant bariatric surgery should be reversible, therefore the Roux-En-Y is recommended. After the weight reaches its nadir, the Roux-En-Y is reversed and abdominoplasty with mesh is performed. In the future, adjuvant bariatric surgery may be completely eliminated by the use of a myointegrated extra-abdominal sequential compression device. Sequential compression decreases intra-abdominal fat volume directly and increases the work of breathing to optimize the rate of weight loss. In the future, plastic surgeons will perform abdominal wall bariatric plastic surgery to cure acquired obesity.

Keywords: Abdominal wall bariatric plastic surgery; Abdominal wall compliance measurements; Biochemical theory of weight regulation; Biomechanical theory of weight regulation; Distribution ratio after liposuction; Intra-abdominal balloon; Intra-abdominal fat transfer; Myointegrated extra-abdominal tissue expander; Obesity and inguinal hernia; Optimizing weight loss; Removal of intra-abdominal fat; Reversible bariatric surgery; Sequential abdominal compression device.

Weight Regulation and Curing Acquired Obesity. https://doi.org/10.1016/B978-0-323-77854-1.00011-1

Additional research can be performed to confirm the neuromechanical hypothesis. Animal experiments, similar to those performed on female brown ground squirrels by Dark et al., can be repeated with removal of only intra-abdominal fat. After intra-abdominal fat removal, meal volume will increase and the increased fat absorbed will be distributed throughout the body. Intra-abdominal fat will be restored to the original fat volume and additional fat volume will be added extra-abdominally, resulting in an increased weight. Weight gain will support the neuromechanical hypothesis of sensing intra-abdominal contents. Animal experiments can also be performed placing an intra-abdominal balloon which increases the value of N. The balloon volume increases tension on the external surface of the stomach which should decrease meal volume resulting in weight loss. The current use of the intragastric balloon is analogous to increasing N. The fat weight equation $O = [(RC_a/Kr_s) - b_aC_a - N]/D$ predicts that increased N will decrease O. Weight loss would support the neuromechanical hypothesis.

Human studies can be performed on women undergoing hysterectomy or oophorectomy for fibroids or large ovarian tumors, respectively. These studies will be similar to those by Carlson. Women routinely have preoperative abdominal scanning used to determine the tumor mass but the scan can also be used to determine intra-abdominal fat volume. After surgical resection and recovery, repeat scanning can be performed to determine intra-abdominal fat volume. The increased volume of intra-abdominal fat should correlate with the volume of the tumor removed. If preoperative whole-body scanning was performed, then the distribution ratio D can be calculated and it would be possible to predict total fat weight. The volume of the tumor removed can be used to calculate the weight gain. A positive correlation supports the N component of the fat weight equation and sensing intra-abdominal contents. A similar human study can be done using whole-body scanning prior to liposuction. After liposuction the distribution ratio D has changed. Repeat scanning should show the same volume of intra-abdominal fat but reduced extra-abdominal fat. Correlation would support the concept of sensing only intra-abdominal fat and the neuromechanical hypothesis.

Recent medical research has shown an inverse relationship of obesity and inguinal hernias.[1] If obesity occurs because of weakness in the anterior abdominal wall, then the incidence of hernias is expected to increase, not decrease. Is this evidence against the hypothesis that physiologic acquired obesity occurs from weakened anterior abdominal wall? Hernias occur with coughing, sneezing, and straining, which are all associated with transient spikes in intra-abdominal pressure. The combination of increased intra-abdominal pressure and the decreased mechanical strength of the anterior abdominal wall creates herniation. Obesity stretches the anterior abdominal muscles and by Starling's law, the muscles have decreased mechanical strength. Since coughing, sneezing, and abdominal straining require strong anterior abdominal wall muscle contraction, then decreased muscle strength would create smaller transient spikes in intra-abdominal pressure. Clinical studies of intra-abdominal pressure in obese people during coughing, sneezing, and straining need to be performed. If obese people did not achieve transient spikes in intra-abdominal pressure comparable to normal weight people, this could explain the decreased incidence of hernia. Then the inverse relationship could not be used to discredit the hypothesis that physiologic acquired obesity is due to mechanical failure of the anterior abdominal wall.

In the future, it may be possible to distinguish irreversible obesity from reversible obesity based on abdominal wall compliance measurements. Compliance calculations are currently available for the lung from the volume and pressure curves. It may be possible to determine compliance by volume pressure measurements using intra-abdominal insufflation similar to that used in laparoscopic surgery. Compliance values could distinguish reversible from irreversible obesity and be used to direct therapy. Diet, exercise, meme changes, and less invasive procedures are effective in reversible obesity, but irreversible obesity requires more aggressive surgical intervention to reinforce the anterior abdominal wall.

The future of curing acquired obesity will be based on reversing the specific pathological component in the neuromechanical model. Currently, liposuction with discarding fat has been used to decrease the denominator in the distribution ratio. Fat transfer to the breasts or buttocks (Brazilian butt lift) for breast or buttocks enhancement, respectively, has grown increasingly popular. In the future, it may be possible to transfer extra-abdominal fat intra-abdominally laparoscopically, possibly in the preperitoneal space. Not all transferred fat survives, but the increase in the numerator of the surviving fat and decrease in the denominator of the nonsurviving fat will increase the distribution ratio. Increasing the distribution ratio increases the feedback, resulting in weight reduction. It may be possible for women to increase their distribution ratio comparable to that of men. This technique may be applicable for female to male gender reassignment or used prophylactically on women having hysterectomy, or removal of any large intra-abdominal mass to prevent weight gain. This technique may also be applicable to normal or over-weight weight patients that intend to reduce weight and redistribute fat for esthetic benefits. It is possible that reversible obesity patients could benefit if the anterior abdominal wall has the mechanical strength necessary to hold the increased intra-abdominal mechanical load. This technique would not be effective initially in irreversible obesity but maybe applicable after abdominal wall reinforcement with mesh.

The alternative to abdominoplasty with mesh reinforcement is a myointegrated extra-abdominal tissue expander. The tissue expander is an adjustable balloon that is placed within the abdominal wall superficial to the muscles and is percutaneously injected to increase volume. Myointegration prevents the balloon from extending outward but compresses on anterior abdominal wall inward. Expansion of the balloon decreases the volume of the abdominal cavity, resulting in increased pressure. For example, if the balloon reduces the abdominal cavity by 1 L, then intra-abdominal fat would have to decrease by 1 L to compensate. If the distribution ratio D is 0.2, then 1 L of intra-abdominal fat reduction results in 5 L of total fat or 10 lbs. reduction. Sequential abdominal compression would ratchet the abdominal cavity progressively smaller, analogous to a reversed pregnancy. A secondary benefit would be that the increased intra-abdominal pressure, and decreased compliance of the anterior abdominal wall, increases the work of breathing. Increasing the caloric expenditure can create the caloric deficit necessary to achieve weight loss. Since the balloon is adjustable, it may be possible to optimize the rate of weight loss based on pulmonary capacity. After the desired weight is achieved, the expander is removed along with the extra skin, then mesh is applied similar to a routine abdominoplasty with mesh reinforcement. The mesh reinforces the weakened anterior abdominal wall, reducing the abdominal wall compliance and abdominal capacity to maintain the reduced weight. Although both tissue expanders and mesh have been approved by the FDA, their combined use for weight reduction has not been approved. This will require a clinical trial monitored by an institutional review board.

The future surgical treatment for acquired irreversible obesity may require a series of two or three operations, dependent on the severity of obesity. The current restrictive and malabsorptive bariatric surgical procedures create abnormal physiology which results in weight loss but also has undesirable side effects. Patients should not suffer a lifetime of complications from a bariatric operation that ceased reducing weight after 2 years. A reversible, restrictive, or malabsorptive bariatric surgical procedure is required for the first stage in all cases. The Roux-en-Y is reversible, but the gastric sleeve is not and therefore is not recommended. After the patients reach their nadir, which usually occurs in less than 2 years, the Roux-en-Y should be reversed. When the BMI is reduced to less than 35, abdominal wall reinforcement with reversal of the bariatric surgery would be performed in the second stage. More severe acquired obesity, with BMI still greater than 35, may require a second-stage placement of a sequential abdominal compression device and reversal of the bariatric surgical procedure. At the third stage, the sequential compression device is removed and replaced with mesh reinforcement.

The last future alternative to consider is eliminating intra-abdominal restrictive and malabsorptive bariatric surgery entirely. The anterior abdominal wall would be evaluated with scans to assess the fat layer thickness, the volume of fat, and to determine the presence of abdominal wall hernias. The first operation consists of liposuction of the anterior abdominal wall to decrease the thickness to approximately 5 cm, which is essential in order to safely perform the second operation. The second operation consists of placement of a sequential abdominal compressive device, resection of the excess hanging skin, resection of the umbilicus, and the repair of any hernias. Sequential abdominal compression optimizes weight loss by increasing the work of breathing. When the desired weight is achieved, the sequential abdominal compressive device is removed, mesh is placed, and any excessive fat or skin is resected. The advantages of these procedures are that the abdominal cavity is not entered, the complications of the restrictive or malabsorptive surgeries are eliminated, and the amount and rate of weight loss is controlled. In the future, plastic surgeons will perform abdominal wall bariatric plastic surgery to cure acquired obesity.

The obesity epidemic has not been curtailed despite extensive medical research and funding. Obesity cannot be cured with empirical treatments without knowledge of weight regulation physiology. The current biochemical theories of weight regulation are based on blood transmission of biochemicals representative of the total fat that activate receptors in the hypothalamus to create satiety. Dr. Koopman's study published in 1985 disproved the blood transmission theory, yet research remains focused on biochemistry. The pharmaceutical industry is a major source of funds for obesity research and it is understandable that they would want to find a biochemical cure. On the other hand, surgical research receives relatively little funding and new procedures cannot be patented. Medical entrepreneurs are drawn to biochemistry not surgery. Research and funding needs redirection to the biomechanical theory of weight regulation.

Reference

1. Rosemar A, Angeras U, Rosengren A. Body mass index and groin hernia 1 34-year follow-up study in Swedish men. *Ann Surg.* 2008;247(6):1064−1068.

Conclusions

12

Abstract

Weight is regulated indirectly by a dual negative feedback control system. The control system depends on multiple components, but failure of two produces physiologic acquired obesity. Mechanical failure of the muscle and fascia of the anterior abdominal wall results in increased abdominal capacity and increased wall compliance. Physiologic acquired obesity becomes irreversible after the fascia is stretched beyond its elastic modulus. Empirical restrictive or malabsorptive bariatric surgery does not reverse wall mechanical failure, but plastic bariatric surgery does. The other cause of acquired obesity occurs within the control system, when the cerebral cortex fails to respond appropriately to the satiety signal generated by the hypothalamus. Man is unique among species and eating for pleasure after satiety has been achieved is an abnormal meme that must be eliminated. Curing acquired obesity requires restoring normal abdominal wall physiology and restoring the normal satiety meme.

Keywords: Abdominoplasty with mesh; Fat volume equation; High fat volume density; Mechanical failure equation; Meme acquired obesity; Myointegrated sequential abdominal compression device; Neuromechanical hypothesis; Physiologic acquired obesity; Restrictive and malabsorptive bariatric surgery; Reverse pregnancy; Satiety equation; Scientific method.

The clinical observation was made that abdominoplasty with mesh reinforcement resulted in weight loss. Scientific method was used to generate a hypothesis for weight regulation. Complex problems frequently require a multidisciplinary approach. Mathematics, physics, control system engineering, anatomy, physiology, and pathology were used to derive the neuromechanical dual closed loop control system model Fig. 12.1. This model was described in detail in Chapter 5 and is summarized as

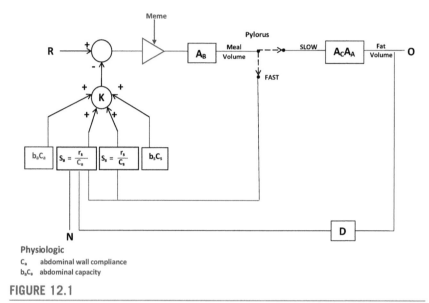

FIGURE 12.1

Physiologic and meme acquired obesity.

follows. Weight is regulated by a control system when caloric intake is greater than or equal to caloric expenditure. There are two cycles, fast and slow, which correlate with the dual closed loops. The fast cycle begins with eating and ends when food is transferred from the stomach to the intestines through the pyloric valve. The fast cycle determines meal volume which is inversely related to fat volume. The satiety equation $M = C_1 - C_2O$ was derived in Appendix 5.1. The slow cycle determines total fat volume which depends on multiple factors including abdominal capacity and compliance. Satiety is achieved in the hypothalamus when the feedback volume exceeds the internal reference volume, which should cause the cortex to terminate the meal. The neuromechanical dual closed loop control system hypothesis is supported by multiple animal experiments and human studies as described in Chapter 6. Of particular importance is Dr. Koopman's experiment using one-way cross-intestinal transfer. His results clinically demonstrate an inverse relationship between meal volume and total fat volume as predicted by the hypotheses.

After developing a weight regulation model, it is possible to mathematically analyze it and determine how component failure could result in acquired obesity. As shown in Fig. 5.3, there are three divisions: neuro, neuromechanical, and mechanical. Analogies to electromechanical control systems, the correlation of pregnancy with obesity and the clinical observation of fascial separation in the anterior abdominal wall, Fig. 4.1, support the concept that physiologic acquired obesity occurs secondary to mechanical failure of the anterior abdominal wall. The mechanical failure cycle, Fig. 8.3, begins with decreased mechanical strength of the anterior abdominal wall. This requires increased intra-abdominal fat volume to achieve satiety, which produces additional stretching of the muscle and fascia, resulting in further loss of wall strength. This cycle repeats and obesity occurs from fat accumulation. Irreversible obesity occurs when the elastic modulus of the fascia is exceeded, resulting in fascial tears. Decreased mechanical strength results in increased compliance C_a and capacity $-b_aC_a$. Weight increases based on the formula derived from Fig. 5.6, $O = [(RC_a/Kr_s) - b_aC_a - N]/D$. Appendix 5.2.

The second cause of acquired obesity is failure to terminate eating when satiety is achieved. Satiety is physiologically determined by the control system, but cortical response is not. Every individual has acquired cultural information that is spread from person to person and establishes their meme. An example of meme-induced acquired obesity was described in Chapter 8. When young Cameroonian men come of age, they follow the cultural tradition of overeating to induce obesity, called guru. Memes of society today differ from those in the past. High fat volume density foods are now readily available worldwide and desirable. Eating beyond satiety for pleasure is so prevalent today that it has become an acceptable meme. Meme changes have contributed to the worldwide epidemic of acquired obesity.

In meme acquired obesity, eating beyond satiety produces mechanical failure of the abdominal wall and the failure cycle begins. These changes are identical to physiological acquired obesity. Unfortunately, physiological acquired obesity may result in frustration and eating beyond satiety, creating a new meme. Although we have described physiologic and meme acquired obesity as two separate etiologies, we have shown that memes can generate physiologic changes, and physiologic changes can generate obesity memes.

The first steps to cure the worldwide epidemic of acquired obesity are education, low fat volume density diet, core exercises when possible, and reversing, when present, the meme of eating beyond satiety. The specific treatment for acquired obesity depends on the pathological type. Reversible obesity may also require surgical therapy including liposuction and abdominoplasty with mesh. Irreversible obesity always requires surgical therapy. In the past, irreversible obesity was treated based on empirical evidence since the physiology of weight regulation and the pathology of acquired obesity was unknown. Weight loss after gastric restriction or intestinal bypass is the basis of the current restrictive and malabsorptive bariatric surgical techniques. These operations are most effective in reducing weight within the first 2 years, but unfortunately produce lifetime complications. Since the restrictive and malabsorption bariatric surgery do not reverse the pathological changes of acquired obesity, Fig. 9.2, these techniques are adjuvants, not cures.

Curing irreversible acquired obesity requires therapy directed at the physiological causes and pathological changes, increased compliance and capacity of the abdomen. Acquired irreversible obesity frequently results in intra-abdominal fat accumulation that usually cannot be reversed by a single operation that increases abdominal wall strength and decreases intra-abdominal volume. The current alternative is to use traditional bariatric surgery as adjuvant and then perform abdominal wall reinforcement at the weight nadar. The other alternative is to perform a series of abdominal wall reinforcements with mesh to ratchet the abdominal cavity smaller. In the future, placing a myointegrated sequential abdominal wall compression device (reverse pregnancy), followed by removal and abdominoplasty with mesh may be available.

The neuromechanical model requires satiety to terminate eating, which is controlled by the cortex. Man is unique and cortical decisions are made by the mind. Our minds contain the memes that have evolved in our culture. Each individual is capable to choosing to respond to satiety or ignore it. The mind can choose between the instant gratification from the pleasure of food verse the delayed gratification of avoiding weight gain and eventual obesity. The neuromechanical weight control system evolved from our DNA and now can be surgically modified, but our memes have ultimate control over our response to satiety and must change to cure acquired obesity.

Index

'Note: Page numbers followed by "f" indicate figures, and "t" indicate tables'

Printed and bound by CPI Group (UK) Ltd, Croydon, CR0 4YY

03/10/2024

01040300-0016